MCQs, MEQs and OSPEs in Occupational Medicine

This second edition of the well-regarded *Multiple Choice Questions and Revision Aid in Occupational Medicine* continues as a comprehensive revision and study resource for those preparing for professional examinations in occupational health, occupational medicine and occupational health and safety.

The content has been extensively revised and updated to cover relevant and current issues. There are three sections organised by question type: MCQ, MEQ and OSPE. Each question is accompanied by the correct answer along with a brief justification where appropriate. The subject topics cover typical occupational health/medicine syllabuses associated with professional examinations, including the use of the 'best of many' MCQ format. The book is essential reading for medical and non-medical practitioners studying for these examinations and will also be useful to those already in the multidisciplinary field or those intending to enter it.

MasterPass Series

100 Medical Emergencies for Finals
Prasanna Sooriakumaran, Channa Jayasena, Anjla Sharman

300 Essential SBAs in Surgery: With Explanatory Answers
Kaji Sritharan, Samia Ijaz, Neil Russel

Cases for Surgical Finals: SAQs, EMQs and MCQs
Philip Stather, Helen Cheshire

Dermatology Postgraduate MCQs and Revision Notes
James Halpern

The Final FRCA Short Answer Questions: A Practical Study Guide
Elizabeth Combeer

Advanced ENT training: A guide to passing the FRCS (ORL-HNS) examination
Joseph Manjaly, Peter Kullar

The Final FRCR: Self-Assessment
Amanda Rabone, Benedict Thomson, Nicky Dineen, Vincent Helyar, Aidan Shaw

Geriatric Medicine: 300 Specialist Certificate Exam Questions
Shibley Rahman, Henry Woodford

Clinical Cases for the FRCA: Key Topics Mapped to the RCoA Curriculum
Alisha Allana

MCQs, MEQs and OSPEs in Occupational Medicine: A Revision Aid
Ken Addley

For more information about this series please visit: www.routledge.com/MasterPass/book-series/CRCMASPASS

MCQs, MEQs and OSPEs in Occupational Medicine

A Revision Aid

Second Edition

Edited by

Ken Addley OBE
Consultant Occupational Physician
Honorary Visiting Professor
Ulster University Business School
Belfast, Northern Ireland

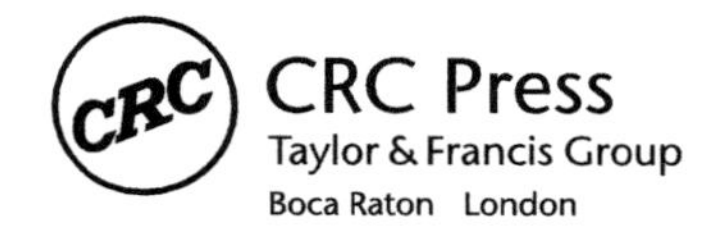

CRC Press is an imprint of the
Taylor & Francis Group, an **informa** business

Second edition published 2023
by CRC Press
6000 Broken Sound Parkway NW, Suite 300, Boca Raton, FL 33487–2742

and by CRC Press
4 Park Square, Milton Park, Abingdon, Oxon, OX14 4RN

CRC Press is an imprint of Taylor & Francis Group, LLC

First edition published 1995 by Taylor & Francis

ISBN: 978-1-032-27240-5 (hbk)
ISBN: 978-1-032-27239-9 (pbk)
ISBN: 978-1-003-29193-0 (ebk)

DOI: 10.1201/9781003291930

Typeset in Helvetica Neue
by Apex CoVantage, LLC

CONTENTS

INTRODUCTION

This second edition of the popular *Multiple Choice Questions and Revision Aid in Occupational Medicine*, with over 500 questions, has been updated and enhanced to include a new offering of traditional multiple choice questions (MCQs), best match and questions in the best of five/best fit format. Also new is the inclusion of modified essay questions (MEQs) and observed structured practical examination questions (OSPEs). In addition, the areas of critical appraisal and report writing are covered within the question sets. These major changes have made the publication both current and relevant to the examinations of diploma, associateship and membership of the Faculty of Occupational Medicine (UK) and licentiateship and membership of Faculty of Occupational Medicine (Royal College of Physicians of Ireland).

An experienced team of occupational and respiratory medicine physicians has brought a wide range of occupational health and medical experience to the compilation of the questions. These contributions encompass academia as well as day-to-day frontline occupational health (OH) practice. The aim of the book is not solely bespoke to the aforementioned examinations but also acts a revision aid and self-assessment reference text for those occupational health nurses, doctors and health and safety professionals studying for other professional occupational health and safety examinations or indeed anyone who has an interest in this field. Realising this aim is achieved by offering a broad range of question types and topics thereby combining self-test with revision and learning.

Occupational medicine has established itself as an important specialty and plays a crucial role in protecting the health, safety and well-being of workers globally. It has become increasingly relevant not least because of the extensive health and safety legislation in place but also as a result of the health and safety response required to manage occupational aspects of the COVID-19 pandemic. The OH specialty has many entering at various levels of involvement and from multidisciplinary backgrounds. The wide variety of questions presented in this book encompasses the broad field of occupational medicine making the book a valuable method of learning, testing knowledge, revision and prompting areas for further exploration and learning.

Finally, I want to thank my panel of expert contributors for putting together what is an up-to-date and comprehensive collection of testing questions.

Ken Addley OBE
Belfast

EDITOR BIOGRAPHY

Professor Ken Addley OBE
MB MD FFOM Hon (UK) FFOM (I) FRCPI

Consultant Occupational Physician with over 25 years' experience in the field of occupational medicine. Academic publishing portfolio includes a range of peer-reviewed medical journal articles, author of the first edition of *Multiple Choice Questions and Revision Aid in Occupational Medicine*, editor of a published textbook on occupational stress and a contributor of chapters in several published occupational medical textbooks.

Awarded an OBE in the Queen's Birthday Honours List 2015 for services to occupational health. Job roles: formerly Director of the Occupational Health Service (OHS) and Centre for Workplace Health Improvement for the Northern Ireland Civil Service. Honorary Visiting Professor in the Ulster University Business School, Belfast.

Fellow of the Faculty of Occupational Medicine, Royal College of Physicians of Ireland and previously Dean, Academic Registrar, National Specialty Director and Research Champion. Annual James Smiley Lecturer and Gold Medal 2016. Visiting Professor to the Faculty of Medicine and Health Sciences, United Arab Emirates University. Awarded a post-graduate doctorate degree (MD) by thesis for research Queen's University Belfast. External Examiner to the Faculty of Medicine, Cardiff University Masters/Diploma course in Occupational Health and External MSc and PhD Thesis Examiner to the Faculty of Medicine, University of Malaysia. ICOH Service Award 2018 as Chair of Scientific Committee, ICOH Triennial Congress, Dublin 2018. Honorary Fellowship of the Faculty of Occupational Medicine, UK. Fellowship of the Royal College of Physicians of Ireland. Other posts: Chairman, Honorary Secretary and Treasurer of the Northern Ireland Group of the Society of Occupational Medicine. Interests include research, employee mental health and stress, corporate health and well-being.

CONTRIBUTORS

Professor John Gallagher MMedSc FFOM FRCPI

Specialist and Clinical Senior Lecturer in Occupational Medicine and Adjunct Professor at University College Cork (UCC). He is a Fellow of the Faculty of Occupational Medicine, Fellow of the Royal College of Physicians of Ireland and Academic Director of the Diploma and Certificate Courses in Safety, Health and Welfare at Work in UCC. He was previously Dean, Vice Dean, National Specialty Director, Specialist Trainer and Examiner with the Faculty of Occupational Medicine, Royal College of Physicians of Ireland. He is a Consultant in Occupational Medicine with the Occupational Health Departments of the Health Service Executive South, Bon Secours Hospital, Mercy and South Infirmary/Victoria Hospitals and Mater Private Hospital, Cork. He is founder and Chief Medical Officer of Cognate Health Ltd. He is also a supervisor and past External Examiner at Cardiff University (UK) MSc programme in OH.

Professor Blánaid Hayes, MB, FRCPI, FFOM, MD

Consultant Occupational Physician and Honorary Clinical Associate Professor (RCSI). Hon Fellow Faculty of Occupational Medicine (UK); Hon Member Society of Occupational Medicine (UK). Robert Mayne Medal: October 2017; Ferguson-Glass Oration: Sydney, May 2018; ICOH Service Award 2018. Fellow of the Royal College of Physicians of Ireland (FRCPI), former Dean of the Faculty of Occupational Medicine (FFOM) and former president of the Irish Society of Occupational Medicine (ISOM). Occupational physician in the health sector for three decades and an advisor to the manufacturing industry. Involved in specialist training in occupational medicine as a supervisor and as National Specialty Director. Contributed to the development of national guidelines on MRSA, hand hygiene and blood-borne viruses. Her research interests include doctors' well-being, needlestick injury and immunisation in healthcare workers.

Dr Martin Hogan MB FRCPI FFOM

Consultant Occupational Physician. Past Dean Faculty of Occupational Medicine, RCPI 2010–2012. Currently Vice-President of ICOH; President ICOH Triennial Congress 2018. National Specialty Director, FOM RCPI 2008–2010. LFOM/MFOM Examiner, FOM RCPI. Annual Jack Eustace Lecture 2010, FOM RCPI, Dublin. His special interests include toxicology, environmental medicine and occupational cancer.

Dr Conor McDonnell MB MICGP FFOMI

Consultant in Occupational Medicine, Health Service Executive. Course Principal of the Distance Learning Course in Occupational Medicine jointly run by the Faculty of Occupational Medicine, Ireland, and the Irish College of General Practitioners. Member of the Examinations Committee of the Faculty of Occupational Medicine. He is a Royal College of Physicians of Ireland trainer for the Occupational Medicine Higher Specialist Training Scheme. He is a past member of the Board of the Faculty of Occupational Medicine. His special interests include remote medicine, workforce planning, work-related stress, sickness absence management, research and teaching.

Dr Paul McKeagney MB MSc (Occ Health) MRCP (Resp) FFOM FRCP

Consultant Respiratory Physician in the Regional Respiratory Centre, Belfast City Hospital. Fellow of Faculty of Occupational Medicine RCPI and Faculty Board Member; Tutor Cardiff University MSc Occupational Health Course; Specialist Interests in COPD and Occupational Lung Disease; Member GORDS UK panel.

Dr David Mills MB BCh MBA MFOM (UK) FFOM (I) FRCPI

Accredited specialist in Occupational Medicine from 2007. Medical Officer in NICS Occupational Service until 2019, the last two years as acting medical director. Currently deputy senior medical officer in the not-for-profit OH provider BHSF. Current board member in Faculty of Occupational Medicine RCP in Dublin. Previous board member of Faculty of Occupational Medicine London (UK).

chapter 01

DOI: 10.1201/9781003291930-01

Multiple Choice Questions (MCQs)

Aviation and Diving

Q1. In aviation medicine, which one of the following statements is true?

a. The air temperature decreases roughly 1°C per thousand feet of ascent.
b. There is a linear decrease in pressure with elevation from sea level.
c. Commercial divers are usually advised to delay flights 24 hours after their last dive to avoid the risk of decompression sickness (DCS).
d. At 15,000 metres above sea level, oxygen has dropped to 15%.
e. Commercial aircraft are usually pressurised to the equivalent of 2,000 feet when travelling at 20,000–30,000 feet in flight.

Q2. In relation to aviation and the Earth's atmosphere, which one of the following statements is the best fit?

a. The stratosphere is the atmospheric layer furthest away from the Earth.
b. Hypoxia arising at increasing altitude is a direct consequence of changes in oxygen concentration.
c. Alveolar oxygen tension falls below 60 mmHg above 10,000 feet.
d. With every 1,000 feet ascent, the temperature drops by 1°C.
e. Military aircraft confine their activities to the tropospheric layer.

Q3. Regarding hypoxia in relation to aviation, which one of the following statements is the best fit?

a. The effects of acute hypoxia can be insidious with visual and mild psychomotor impairment.
b. Oxygen enrichment of air supply mitigates the risk of hypoxia.
c. Military aircraft are pressurised to the same degree as commercial aircraft.
d. Cognitive impairment may occur at levels of 8,000–10,000 feet.
e. Sensorimotor impairment may occur at levels of 8,000–10,000 feet.

Q4. Which one of the following is the best fit as the most common medical reason for grounding air crew?

a. Ear, nose and throat.
b. Cardiovascular.
c. Psychiatric.
d. Musculoskeletal.
e. Neurological.

Q5. In diving medicine and decompression sickness (DCS), which one of the following statements is the best fit?

a. Pulmonary syndrome symptoms of DCS tend to occur in isolation of other DCS features.
b. 'The chokes' occurs in at least 20% of DCS cases.

c. Recompression results in quick reversal of pulmonary symptoms in most cases.
d. Although quite painful and distressing, pulmonary syndrome in DCS is unlikely to be fatal.
e. Classical pulmonary syndrome is accompanied by tachypnoea, cyanosis and hypertension.

Q6. In regard to decompression sickness, which one of the following statements is correct?

a. Nitrogen enters and leaves fat tissue more rapidly than oxygen or carbon dioxide.
b. Osteonecrosis occurs in a small proportion of divers.
c. Symptoms are due to oxygen and carbon dioxide bubble formation.
d. Results from the physiologic effects of toxic gases.
e. Aseptic necrosis typically involves the head or shaft of the humerus.

Q7. For limb pain associated with decompression sickness, which one of the following is the best fit?

a. Affects large and small joints equally.
b. Is significantly aggravated by moving the affected joint.
c. If not symptomatic within one hour is unlikely to occur.
d. Limb pain not localised to a joint may be due to swelling of a muscle.
e. Arises from the formation of gas micro-bubbles which had been dissolved in body tissues according to Boyle's law.

Q8. When immersed upright in water, which one of the following effects does NOT occur?

a. Left atrial pressure rises.
b. Blood volume in the chest increases.
c. Blood from the lower extremities is forced upwards.
d. Diuresis.
e. Carbon dioxide retention.

Biological Hazards, Biological Monitoring and Vaccinations

Q9. In regard to SARS-CoV-2 virus, which one of the following is the best fit?

a. Is a DNA virus.
b. Is an RNA virus.
c. Is commonly associated with increased adverse outcome in pregnancy.
d. Is most commonly transmitted by aerosols.
e. Transmission by fomites is common.

Q10. After allowance for other factors, which one of the following does NOT carry any material increase in risk of an individual developing serious or fatal COVID-19?

a. Smoking status.
b. Ethnicity.
c. Age.
d. Body mass index greater than 30 kg/m^2.
e. Gender.

Q11. In biological hazard groups under Control of Substances Hazardous to Health UK 2002 (COSHH) regulations, which one of the following statements is the best fit?

a. Group 1 pathogens cause human disease but are easily treated.
b. A new biological agent can be assumed to start in Group 1.
c. Group 4 biological agents usually cause severe human illness with no treatment or prophylaxis available.
d. The Advisory Committee on Dangerous Pathogens UK (ACDP) advises on human and animal pathogens.
e. The approved list does not contain genetically modified organisms.

Q12. Needlestick (and other sharps) injuries (NSIs) in healthcare are considered to be largely preventable. Which one of the following statements is the best fit?

a. There is good evidence that specific legislation (e.g., US 2006 and EU 2013) reduces the incidence of NSIs.
b. There is good evidence that safety engineered devices (i.e., engineering controls) are the most effective intervention to prevent NSIs.
c. Prevention of NSIs is best achieved by providing regular training in sharps safety to ensure compliance with 'Standard Precautions'.
d. More than 25 blood-borne viruses have been reported following NSIs in healthcare and laboratory workers.
e. The risk of acquiring hepatitis C from a freshly contaminated hollow-bore needle is of the order of 1/300.

Q13. Which one of the following statements is incorrect in regard to brucellosis?

a. Brucella are small, gram-negative, aerobic coccobacilli.
b. There are three species of public health significance: *Melitensis*, *Abortus*, *Suis*.
c. *Abortus* is the most pathogenic and invasive species.
d. Animal-to-human transmission is mainly via contaminated or untreated milk or milk products.
e. The onset of illness can be insidious or abrupt.

Q14. Which one of the following statements is incorrect?

a. Q fever is caused by infection with *Coxiella burnetii*.
b. Orf is a parapoxvirus.
c. Lyme disease is caused by the spirochaete *Borrelia burgdorferi*.
d. Anthrax is caused by the gram-negative bacteria *Bacillus anthracis*.
e. Ringworm is a common fungal infection of the skin.

Q15. In regard to Lyme disease, which one of the following statements is incorrect?

a. Lyme disease is a parapoxvirus.
b. It is a disease of exacerbations and remissions.
c. It often begins with a flu-like illness.
d. It is associated with a characteristic skin lesion: erythema migrans.
e. It may involve joints, the nervous system or heart.

Q16. Which one of the following statements is incorrect?

a. Anthrax is caused by the gram-positive bacteria *Bacillus anthracis*.
b. *Bacillus anthracis* spores have a short viability.
c. *Bacillus anthracis* can be transmitted by cutaneous contact.
d. *Bacillus anthracis* can be transmitted by inhalation.
e. *Bacillus anthracis* can be transmitted via the gastrointestinal system.

Q17. Standard and Transmission-Based Precautions are key to minimising the spread of infection in the healthcare environment. In regard to Standard Precautions, which one of the following statements is NOT in line with these guidelines?

a. Standard Precautions are basic practices that are applied to the care of patients with known infections.
b. Hand hygiene is an element of Standard Precautions.
c. Respiratory hygiene and cough etiquette are elements of Standard Precautions.
d. Environmental cleaning and disinfection are elements of Standard Precautions.
e. Risk assessment and use of appropriate personal protective equipment are elements of Standard Precautions.

Q18. Standard and Transmission-Based Precautions are key to minimising the spread of infection in the healthcare environment. In regard to Transmission-Based precautions, which one of the following statements is NOT in line with these guidelines?

a. Transmission-Based Precautions are practices that are implemented for the care of patients with documented or suspected infections.
b. Contact precautions are elements of Transmission-Based Precautions.
c. Sharps safety precautions are elements of Transmission-Based Precautions.
d. Droplet precautions are elements of Transmission-Based Precautions.
e. Airborne precautions are elements of Transmission-Based Precautions.

In regard to food poisoning, match the following:

Q19. Salmonella food poisoning.

Q20. *Staphylococcus aureus* food poisoning.

Q21. *Clostridium welchii* food poisoning.

Q22. *Bacillus cerus* food poisoning.

Q23. *Clostridium botulinum* food poisoning.

a. Toxin. Spore-producing organism. Onset of symptoms within 1 to 16 hours. Associated with fried rice.
b. Toxin. Can be rapidly fatal. Onset of symptoms within 18 to 36 hours.
c. Onset of symptoms within 2–6 hours. Organism found in skin folds, nasal passages and septic skin lesions.
d. Onset of symptoms within 2 to 72 hours. Biggest single cause of food poisoning in the UK. Associated with poultry and poultry products.
e. Enterotoxin: onset of symptoms within 8 to 24 hours. Anaerobic organism.

In regard to food hygiene, match the following:

Q24. Conditions for bacterial growth.

Q25. Risk factors when controlling contamination.

Q26. Assessment of food handlers.

Q27. Action following outbreak of food poisoning.

Q28. Ideal factory or kitchen environments.

a. Condition of raw food and hygiene of handlers. Cleanliness of kitchens and equipment. Conditions for food storage.
b. Exclude infectious diseases. Investigate diarrhoeal illness. Disqualify active and persistent infective discharges from ears, nose and eyes.
c. Notify public health department, identify affected persons and source for analysis. Share information with environmental health officers, local hospitals, laboratories and general practitioners.
d. Clean the premises/machinery with adequate ventilation and waste disposal. Separate cloakroom facilities. Maintained refrigerators/chillers for food storage.
e. Suitable food medium and temperature. Adequate moisture and sufficient time.

In regard to these biological agents, match the following:

Q29. Anthrax (*Bacillus anthracis*).

Q30. Leptospirosis.

Q31. Brucellosis (*Brucella abortus*).

Q32. Hepatitis B (HBV).

Q33. Legionellosis (*Legionella pneumophilia*).

a. Contracted from infected bovine carcasses or ingesting raw milk.
b. Occurs in outbreaks. Associated with cooling towers and air conditioning systems.
c. From infected blood or blood products. Needlestick injury an important occupational factor.
d. Handling of wool, hides and carcasses of infected animals. Two forms: cutaneous and pulmonary.
e. Flu-like illness with jaundice. Involves contact with urine of rodents, dogs or bovines.

Q34. A healthcare worker presents with the following hepatitis B serology results:

- HBsAg Positive.
- HBeAg Negative.
- Anti-HBc IgM Weak Positive/Negative.
- Anti-HBc Total Positive.
- Anti-HBs Negative.

Which one of the following is the correct interpretation of these results?

a. Susceptibility to HBV.
b. Acute HBV infection.

c. HBeAg negative chronic HBV infection.
d. Resolved HBV infection.
e. Response to HBV vaccine.

Q35. Concerning hepatitis B, which one of the following statements is the best fit?

a. Healthcare workers (HCWs) with an anti-HBs response of less than 100 mIU/ml after full vaccination should be regarded as non-responders.
b. HCWs with positive HBeAg cannot perform exposure prone procedures (EPPs) regardless of HBV DNA levels.
c. Hepatitis B vaccines are not live vaccines and can be given to immunosuppressed workers, though their response may be impaired.
d. Public Health England continues to monitor significant occupational exposures to blood-borne viruses and their regular report. Eye of the Needle continues to record one or two hepatitis B seroconversions per year in the UK.
e. HCWs who refuse hepatitis B vaccination or are non-responders cannot work where they would perform EPPs.

Q36. When assessing tuberculosis (TB) as an occupational infection, which one of the following statements is the best fit?

a. Interferon gamma release assay (IGRA) tests that measure the B-cell specific Y-interferon release to TB antigens have transformed detection of latent TB in the UK.
b. Even though the evidence shows BCG is ineffective after the age of 35, it continues to be recommended on a precautionary basis for healthcare workers at risk.
c. In a case of TB in a long-haul flight aircraft crew member, passengers are not routinely contact traced though other members of staff may be.
d. Detecting latent TB is critical as 35% will convert to active TB disease and the majority of conversion is in the first two years.
e. Documentary evidence of BCG and/or a scar in an asymptomatic person is adequate to pass pre-placement TB screening in a healthcare worker.

Q37. In regard to tuberculosis (TB) and IGRA, which one of the following statements is incorrect?

a. The immune response to *Mycobacterium tuberculosis* is a cell-mediated immune response.
b. T-cells are sensitised to *Mycobacterium tuberculosis* antigens.
c. Activated effector T-cells produce a cytokine called interferon gamma when stimulated by the *Mycobacterium tuberculosis* antigens.
d. A negative IGRA test result rules out latent TB infection.
e. A negative IGRA test result rules out active TB infection.

Q38. Which one of the following procedures is NOT an exposure prone procedure (EPP)?

a. Oral surgical procedures.
b. Episiotomy.
c. Rectal or vaginal examination in the presence of suspected pelvic trauma.
d. Insertion and maintenance of arterial or intravenous cannulae whether inserted centrally or peripherally.
e. Insertion of intercostal catheter, where the procedure requires insertion of a finger into the pleural cavity in a trauma situation.

Q39. In relation to psittacosis, which one of the following is the best fit?

a. Is caused by *Chlamydophylia ornitii*.
b. Is usually treated with penicillins.
c. The incubation period is one to four weeks.
d. Is most frequently transmitted to humans by budgies.
e. Is a form of hyperimmune response.

Q40. You are employed by a care home to provide occupational health advice for their 100 employees, 80 of whom provide direct clinical care to elderly patients. The manager is keen to implement an annual seasonal influenza vaccination programme for staff to reduce nosocomial influenza. In encouraging staff to engage with the programme, which one of the following statements about influenza and/or vaccination is the best fit?

a. About one-fifth of healthcare workers acquire influenza annually.
b. Influenza vaccination may be trivalent or quadrivalent.
c. Vaccine efficacy in healthy adults typically ranges from 70% to 90%.
d. Vaccine should be used with caution in pregnant women.
e. Vaccine has been shown to reduce the risk of stroke.

Q41. Welders exposed to metal fumes should be immunised against which one of the following biological agents?

a. *Mycobacterium tuberculosis*.
b. *Neisseria meningitidis*.
c. *Varicella zoster*.
d. *Haemophilus influenzae*.
e. *Streptococcus pneumoniae*.

Q42. A worker who works on open hillsides with brambles and scrub is concerned about a tick-borne disease. Which one of the following is the best fit?

a. Malaria.
b. Dengue fever.
c. Leishmaniasis.
d. Lyme disease.
e. Yellow fever.

Q43. Which one of the following statements regarding vaccines in an occupational setting is the best fit?

a. A poor response to hepatitis B vaccination is associated with male gender, obesity, age over 40 and smoking.
b. Monovalent hepatitis A vaccine is a live attenuated vaccine and should not be given in pregnancy.
c. Inactivated quadrivalent influenza vaccination contains antigens from two type A, one type B and one type C strains of the virus.
d. Varicella vaccination is a sub-unit vaccine and may be given in pregnancy.
e. An adult may be considered to have lifelong immunity to tetanus if they have been documented as having had five doses of (toxoid) vaccination.

Q44. Messenger RNA vaccines consist of genetic material (mRNA) that instructs the recipient's antigen-presenting cells to make the identified antigen, thus stimulating an immune response against the virus. For SARS-CoV-2, which one of the following statements does NOT fit?

a. mRNA vaccines encode the spike protein that, when expressed on the cell surface, provokes generation of neutralising antibodies and activation of T-cells.
b. The neutralising antibodies prevent infection by blocking virus fusion with the host cell.
c. The mRNA is encapsulated in a lipid nanoparticle, to facilitate entry into a host cell.
d. Slow degradation of mRNA within cells contributes to the safety profile of these vaccines.
e. mRNA vaccines have a high potency.

Q45. When considering vaccination in occupational health settings, which one of the following statements is the best fit?

a. There is not much evidence available of the effectiveness of BCG after the age of 35, but prior to that the efficacy is 90%.
b. BCG is contraindicated in HIV-positive patients if the viral load is greater than 1,000 cp/m.
c. The lifetime risk of TB disease after testing positive for latent TB is 5% to 10% regardless of whether a person had previous BCG.
d. A person at high contact risk who has no BCG scar but certificate evidence of BCG more than 20 years ago and negative IGRA test can have a BCG.
e. In the UK 75% of TB infection is pulmonary and therefore more infectious.

Q46. In biological monitoring, which one of the following statements does NOT fit?

a. Urinary creatinine levels increase with age.
b. Men have substantially higher levels of urinary creatinine than women.
c. Urinary creatinine levels are typically slightly lower in the afternoon than the morning.
d. Creatinine is the metabolite of creatine, an important energy store for muscles in the form of the creatine phosphate bond.
e. The excretion of creatinine is almost entirely by glomerular filtration in the kidneys.

Q47. When considering biological monitoring for metals, which one of the following statements is the best fit?

a. End-of-shift timing is critical in urine monitoring for mercury.
b. Cobalt is exerted mainly in faeces but biological monitoring is by urine sample.
c. Urine levels of cobalt lower rapidly 24 hours after exposure.
d. Biological monitoring is mainly indicated in skin exposure to toxic metals.
e. Hexavalent chromium biological monitoring is best done with an end-of-shift urine sample.

Q48. In biological monitoring, which one of the following is the best fit?

a. Provides a direct assessment of dermal exposure.
b. Provides an assessment of efficacy of personal protective equipment.
c. Is a measurement of a biological effect in exposed workers.
d. Is not a surrogate of absorbed dose.
e. Is an example of primary prevention.

Q49. Which one of the following is an example of biological effect monitoring?

a. Measurement of lead in urine for lead exposure.
b. Measurement of lead in blood for lead exposure.
c. Measurement of cholinesterase activity for organophosphate exposure.
d. Measurement of hippuric acid in urine for toluene exposure.
e. Measurement of volatile organic compounds in exhaled air.

Q50. When considering biological monitoring for toluene, which one of the following is the best fit?

a. Can be effectively done only with blood samples.
b. o-Cresol in urine should be measured at the end of a shift.
c. Is performed with methyl hippuric acid in urine.
d. Is a form of biological effect monitoring.
e. Is rarely indicated.

Environmental Protection

Q51. Which one of the following health effects of environmental tobacco smoke (ETS) on adults has not been proven?

a. Increased risk of breast cancer in postmenopausal women by 5%.
b. Increased risk of coronary heart disease by 25–30%.
c. Increased risk of lung cancer by 20–30%.
d. Increased risk of stillbirth by 23%.
e. Increased risk of congenital malformation by 13%.

Q52. In sick building syndrome (SBS), which one of the following statements does NOT apply?

a. Chemical air contaminants can include volatile organic compounds (VOCs), tobacco smoke, formaldehyde and inorganic gases chlorine and carbon monoxide.
b. VOCs may evaporate from upholstery, adhesives and carpeting, contributing to SBS.
c. Computers may emit low levels of VOCs, contributing to SBS symptoms.
d. Ozone, hydrocarbons and dust may be emitted from photocopiers.
e. Cross-sectional studies have documented a correlation between airborne particulate concentration and SBS symptoms.

Q53. When assessing potential cardiovascular health outcomes from environmental traffic noise the most appropriate dB noise indicator is:

a. LEX.
b. Lden.
c. Lnight.
d. Lday.
e. LA,max.

Q54. The electromagnetic field around high voltage power lines is which one of the following?

a. Measured in V/m (volt per metre).
b. Significantly above background levels even at 200 m from the lines.

c. Classified as probably carcinogenic by the IARC (International Agency for Research on Cancer).
d. At ground level are typically orders of magnitude greater than those emitted by household electrical items.
e. Measured in µT (Microtesla).

Q55. In relation to environmental protection, which one of the following statements is the best fit?

a. Guideline values in relation to water and/or air safety are based on the concentration of a constituent that results in no significant lifetime risk if consumed.
b. Earth is now in the Anthropocene geological era whereby 'made' materials represent 90% of the volume of living materials.
c. Anthropogenic mass has been growing exponentially since the Industrial Revolution.
d. The well-defined precautionary principle underpins European and international legislation and treaties in relation to environmental protection.
e. An endocrine disrupter is an exogenous substance that causes adverse health effects in an intact organism or its progeny.

Q56. In relation to firefighters exposed to environmental toxins at the World Trade Center (WTC) site on 9/11, which one of the following associations has NOT been described?

a. Increased long-term cardiovascular disease risk is associated with increased WTC exposure.
b. Increased risk of monoclonal gammopathy of undetermined significance, a precursor or multiple myeloma, is associated with increased exposure.
c. Increased incidence of cancers generally when compared with other US firefighters.
d. Increased risk of Barrett's oesophagus is associated with increased WTC exposure.
e. Increased risk of sleep apnoea.

Q57. For environmental protection the precautionary principle is best described as which one of the following statements?

a. Avoid changes in the environment until certain that there will be no deleterious effect.
b. Take all available precautions to protect the environment.
c. Lack of scientific certainty must not be used as a reason to ignore or postpone preventive or remedial action when there are other good reasons to do so.
d. Scientific certainty should be required for remedial actions to ensure further harm is avoided.
e. The driving force for environmental change is precaution.

Epidemiology and Statistics

Q58. Within the Bradford Hill criteria for causal inference, which one of the following is the most persuasive for causality in modern epidemiology?

a. Consistency.
b. Specificity.
c. Temporality.
d. Biological gradient.
e. Plausibility.

Q59. In designing a protocol for a vaccination programme requiring two doses, researchers may choose to report on either or both an 'intention to treat' or a 'per protocol' analysis. Which one of the following statements does NOT fit?

a. All participants who were randomised were included in the intention to treat analysis.
b. Participants who died during the period of exploration were included in the intention to treat analysis.
c. Trial participants who received the intervention but were lost to follow-up were excluded from the intention to treat analysis.
d. The per protocol analysis included only those participants who completed the vaccination schedule.
e. Intention to treat reflects what would usually happen in clinical practice.

Q60. Which one of the following statements on central tendency does NOT fit?

a. The mean, median and mode are measures of central tendency.
b. The mean is the average value.
c. The median is the is the value on the scale that divides the distribution into two equal parts.
d. The mode is the most frequently occurring value.
e. The median of the numbers 3, 8, 2, 4, 7, 8 equals 4.

Q61. A cause of a disease is an event, condition, characteristic or a combination of these factors which plays an important role in producing the disease. Which one of the following types of study has the strongest ability to prove causation?

a. Bradford Hill.
b. Cross-sectional study (also known as prevalence).
c. Case-control study (also known as case-reference).
d. Randomised controlled trial (also known as clinical trial).
e. Cohort study (also known as follow-up).

Q62. Confounding occurs when the effects of two exposures (risk factors) have not been separated and it is therefore incorrectly concluded that the effect is due to one rather than the other variable. Which one of the following methods do NOT control confounding?

a. Randomisation.
b. Restriction.
c. Matching.
d. Stratification.
e. Validity.

Q63. Age-specific cancer incidence rate is defined by which one of the following?

a. Number of new cases of cancer detected in a defined population in a specified period of time.
b. Number of old and new cases of cancer detected in a defined population in a specified period of time.
c. Number of new cases of pre-cancers detected in a defined population in a specified period of time.
d. Number of new cases of cancer detected.
e. Number of cancer patients treated in a 12-month period.

Match the following definitions:

Q64. Sensitivity.

Q65. Specificity.

Q66. Efficiency.

Q67. Validity.

Q68. Repeatability.

a. Representing a true assessment of what it measures and compares with established methods.
b. Detection of a high proportion of true positives.
c. An expression of the extent of agreement between repeated measurements in the same subject under same conditions.
d. Related to the proportion of all subjects tested who have been correctly diagnosed or classified.
e. Detection of a high proportion of false negatives which are classified as negative by a test.

Match the following definitions:

Q69. Prevalence rate.

Q70. Incidence rate.

Q71. Standardised mortality ratio (SMR).

Q72. Odds ratio.

Q73. Proportional mortality ratio.

a. The number of a population at risk who develop a condition within a stated time period.
b. A weighted average of the ratios of age-specific mortality proportions in two groups.
c. A measure of the risk of disease in a study population compared with that of a reference population.
d. The number of a population who have a condition at a given time or over a stated period of time.
e. An age-standardised measure of mortality in a study group relative to that in a reference group.

Match the following definitions:

Q74. Mean.

Q75. Mode.

Q76. Median.

Q77. Frequency distribution curve.

Q78. Normal distribution curve.

a. The value of a variable which has the highest frequency.
b. The sum of all observed values divided by the number of observations.
c. Shows the underlying distribution of a variable in an infinitely large population.
d. Is unimodal, bell-shaped and completely symmetrical about its mean.
e. The middle value of a series of observations placed in either ascending or descending order.

Match the following definitions:

Q79. Standard deviation.

Q80. Standard error.

Q81. Correlation coefficient.

Q82. Confidence intervals.

Q83. Regression coefficient.

a. The variability of sample means in relation to the population value.
b. Indicates the relationship between one set of variables and another using the slope of a line drawn to represent them.
c. A range of values within which a particular statistic value lies.
d. A measure of the dispersion of values about their mean.
e. Measures the strength of a linear relationship between two variables.

Q84. When critically appraising a published paper in a journal, which one of the following types of study design is best used to determine the incidence of a disease?

a. Cross-sectional study.
b. Case-control study.
c. Cohort study.
d. Randomised controlled trial.
e. Periodic sample survey.

Q85. A study is designed to investigate the relative risk of cancer from living within 5 km of an industrial facility. The authors looked at the relative risk of 32 different cancers inside the 5 km distance as compared with the expected rates using the national cancer rates for the country. Relative risks and their 95% confidence intervals (95% CIs) were estimated for all the analyses on the basis of Poisson regression models, using a Bayesian model. Statistical significance was taken if the 95% CIs excluded 1 (unity). Two cancers were identified as having a statistically significant increase. Colorectal cancer had a relative risk of 1.1 with CI of 1.04 to 1.16. Leukaemia was significant in women, but not men, and had an overall relative risk of 1.08 in women with CI of 1.01 to 1.2. The CI for men includes unity. When carrying out a critical appraisal of the findings of the paper, which one of the following statements is the best fit?

a. There is a likelihood of a relationship between colorectal cancers and leukaemia in women and the facility.
b. There is a likelihood of a relationship between colorectal cancers but not leukaemia and the facility.

c. As only 2 cancers of 32 studied were shown to be statistically significant at the chosen level, few inferences can be drawn.
d. The study should be repeated but using local rather than national cancer rates.
e. Poisson regression models are inappropriate in this type of study so renders the study meaningless.

Q86. When critically appraising a systematic review, which one of the following statements is the best fit?

a. In the forest plot the diamond usually represents the most powerful study.
b. Clinical and statistical heterogeneity are essentially the same thing.
c. A funnel plot is very helpful in assessing the power of a systematic review.
d. Using a published search strategy a big database like Medline will be acceptable.
e. The methods for assessing the quality of the studies should be agreed before any literature search begins.

Q87. Considering critical appraisal of a published paper, which one of the following is the best fit?

a. Determine whether the study addressed a clearly focused issue.
b. Identify the study population.
c. Interpret the results.
d. Assess for bias.
e. Determine whether the study can be applied to practice.

Q88. The 'PICO' formulation or model is a useful tool for appraising research publications. In the context of occupational health practice, which one of the following statements does NOT fit?

a. 'P' refers to the population from which the study sample is drawn (e.g., case-control study).
b. 'I' refers to the incidence of a disease/condition in a given population (e.g., cross-sectional study).
c. 'C' refers to the comparison group (i.e., the control group in a case-control study, cohort study or randomised controlled trial).
d. 'O' refers to the outcome in terms of therapeutic response (e.g., randomised controlled trial, systematic review).
e. 'P' refers to the problem (e.g., disease status) or patient.

Fitness for Work, Rehabilitation and Shift Work

Q89. Dizziness represents a major challenge to health professionals. It is common, often becomes chronic and remains largely untreated. Which one of the following statements is incorrect?

a. Peripheral vestibular neuronitis may be considered as an acute reversible peripheral neuropathy.
b. Benign positional vertigo is the most common form of vestibular dizziness.
c. Benign positional vertigo is diagnosed with a Dix–Hallpike test.
d. Vestibular suppressant medication should be restricted to the acute phase of a vestibular episode.
e. Vestibular rehabilitation therapy is of limited use in the treatment for continuous or chronic dizziness.

Q90. Screening for 'yellow flags' can help to identify those workers with low back pain who are at risk of developing chronic pain and disability—Faculty of Occupational Medicine guidelines for the assessment of the worker presenting with low back pain (LBP). Which one of the following is a 'yellow flag'?

a. Age of onset less than 20 years or greater than 55 years.
b. Persisting severe restriction of lumbar spine flexion.
c. An expectation that passive rather than active treatment will be beneficial.
d. Systemically unwell: fever and unexplained weight loss.
e. Widespread neurology.

Q91. Diabetes mellitus is a metabolic disorder characterised by chronic hyperglycaemia due to insulin deficiency or resistance or both. It leads to both microvascular and macrovascular complications. Which one of the following statements is incorrect?

a. HbA1c is a fraction of glycosylated haemoglobin (normal value less than 7%), and its measurement provides an accurate estimate of mean glucose levels over the preceding six months, which correlates with the risk of macrovascular complications.
b. More employees with type 1 diabetes who do shift work experience problems with their jobs compared with controls.
c. A higher rate of sickness absence has been shown to be associated with manual work activity in those with diabetes.
d. Sickness absence is higher in people with diabetes (types 1 and 2) in general.
e. Employees with type 1 diabetes who worked shifts are more likely to have a higher HbA1c, increasing their risk of microvascular complications in the long term.

Q92. Concerning the older worker, which statement is the best fit?

a. The age-dependency ratio has now stabilised after decades of falling.
b. The equality legislation makes it impossible to set a compulsory retirement age.
c. Higher levels of education only minimally affect health in ageing.
d. Between 5% and 20% of people over the age of 65 have mild cognitive impairment.
e. The healthy worker effect is irrelevant.

Q93. In regard to color vision testing using Ishihara plates, which one of the following is correct?

a. Recommended lighting is a Macbeth easel lamp.
b. Should be viewed at 25 cm from the face.
c. Delay of over four seconds in identifying a number can be ignored.
d. One error on plate 2 to 13 of the 24-plate test indicates a color deficit.
e. Testing is performed on both eyes at the same time.

Q94. In relation to the reproductive effects, which one of the following is not a recognised effect of shift work?

a. Subfertility in women.
b. Increased risk of spontaneous abortion.

c. Prematurity.
d. Low birth weight.
e. Menstrual disturbance.

Q95. When considering reproductive disorders, which one of the following statements is the best fit?

a. Data from Public Health England in 2018 would suggest that 7.5% of women have severe reproductive disorders.
b. High-level exposure to carbon disulphide reduces libido in workers.
c. Dental nurses exposed to higher levels of nitrous gas can have increased miscarriage rates and reduced B12 and folate production.
d. Psychological work stress affects female fertility primarily rather than male.
e. The Workplace (Health, Safety and Welfare) Regulations 1990 require an employer to make suitable facilities for pregnant workers to rest, including breast feeding.

Q96. The female reproductive system can be adversely affected by exposure to organic solvents. Which one of the following effects has NOT been reported?

a. Increased risk of spontaneous abortion and congenital malformation.
b. Increased prevalence of menstrual disorders.
c. Increased risk of vaginal adenocarcinoma in offspring of exposed women.
d. Reduced female fertility levels with exposure to high levels of solvents.
e. Increased risk of leukaemia in offspring of exposed women.

Q97. The Disabilities of the Arm, Shoulder and Hand (DASH) questionnaire is used as an indicator of the impact of an impairment on the level and type of disability. In regard to the DASH score, which one of the following statements does NOT fit?

a. The score ranges from 0 *(no disability)* to 100 *(most severe disability)*.
b. It assesses the whole person's ability to function, even if the person is compensating with the other limb.
c. It describes the disability experienced by people with lower limb disorders.
d. It monitors changes in symptoms and function over time.
e. It can detect and differentiate small and large changes of disability over time after surgery.

Q98. Which one of the following factors is NOT associated with an unsuccessful return-to-work (RTW) following a workplace upper limb injury?

a. Greater self-reported functional disability.
b. Baseline depression.
c. Higher mean baseline pain.
d. Lower QuickDASH score.
e. Pain catastrophising.

Q99. Following the diagnosis of an illness, a patient generates an organised pattern of beliefs to cope with it, which in turn influences their behaviour. Health psychologists have called these beliefs 'illness perceptions'. Regarding illness perceptions, which one of the following statements does NOT fit?

a. Patients with the same illness may have different perceptions of their condition and different emotional reactions to it.
b. Employees on sick leave have more negative perceptions about their illness than their occupational physicians.
c. Employees with negative perceptions about their illness are less likely to return to work than those with positive ones.
d. Negative perceptions may be more disabling than the illness and need to be addressed to facilitate an early return to work.
e. Identifying negative perceptions does not cause difficulties in the doctor–patient relationship.

Q100. Upper extremity musculoskeletal disorders (UEMSD) are a significant cause of disability and lost productivity globally. Which one of the following workplace programmes/interventions does NOT fit?

a. Work-based resistance training programmes can help prevent UEMSD and symptoms.
b. Work-based resistance training programmes can help manage UEMSD and symptoms.
c. Job stress management training has no impact on the prevalence of UEMSD and symptoms.
d. EMG biofeedback training has no impact on the prevalence of UEMSD and symptoms.
e. Workstation adjustment alone can reduce the prevalence of UEMSD.

Q101. Epidemics can have a disproportionate impact on healthcare workers who are required to care for ill patients while at the same time cope, on a personal level, with the community and societal impact of these diseases. Which one of the following statements is the best fit?

a. Effective interventions are similar despite a wide range of settings and types of outbreaks.
b. Effective interventions are best customised to account for the unique challenges of particular pathogens, geographic location and culture.
c. Younger healthy workers experience less distress.
d. Levels of stress and psychological distress diminish in line with diminishing disease prevalence.
e. Psychological first aid (PFA) has no clear role in mitigating psychological distress in this context.

Q102. Burnout is a major concern for clinicians and their employers. Regarding interventions, which one of the following statements is the best fit?

a. Mindfulness-based stress reduction (MBSR) programmes reduce burnout.
b. Educational interventions addressing communication skills and self-confidence reduce burnout.
c. Workplace interventions addressing workload and shift patterns with meetings to enhance teamwork reduce burnout.
d. Regular small-group debriefing sessions with exploration of coping mechanisms reduce burnout.
e. Incentivised exercise programmes with teams to improve accountability reduce burnout.

Q103. Which one of the following is NOT a useful tool in the rehabilitation of a worker injured at work?

a. Appropriate financial compensation.
b. Reduced numbers of hours in working day.
c. Reduced number of days in working week.
d. Alternative roles.
e. Use of equipment.

Q104. A 48-year-old woman presents with a three-week history of absence from work with a history of non-radicular low back pain and no history of trauma. X-rays show degenerative changes. When managing the case, which one of the following is the best fit?

a. Bed rest for two weeks.
b. Core muscle strengthening.
c. MRI scan to clarify.
d. A polypropylene body jacket.
e. Referral to a pain specialist.

Q105. According to World Health Organization (WHO) classification, an example of an impairment is which one of the following?

a. Ischaemic brain damage.
b. Weakness of one arm.
c. Loss of ability to get showered.
d. Need for a knee brace to walk.
e. Having a cardiac pacemaker.

Q106. Night workers in the European Union (EU) Regulations are defined by which one of the following?

a. Workers who work only at night-time.
b. Workers who work between the hours of 12 midnight and 6 a.m.
c. Workers who work between the hours of 12 midnight and 7 a.m.
d. Workers who work shift work.
e. Workers who work between the hours of 11 p.m. and 6 a.m.

Q107. When considering shift work, which one of the following is the best fit?

a. Counterclockwise rotation of shifts is generally better tolerated.
b. Is contraindicated in insulin-dependent diabetics.
c. Cardiovascular disorders are the most common health effect.
d. The risk of injury is 30% higher on night shift than on morning shift.
e. Shift work sleep disorder occurs in less than 10% of people.

Q108. The part of the brain that regulates biological rhythms is which one of the following?

a. Suprachiasmatic nucleus.
b. Thalamus.
c. Cerebellum.
d. Pontine nucleus.
e. Neocortex.

Q109. When considering who best tolerates shift work, which one of the following is the best fit?

a. Men.
b. Older, experienced workers.
c. Introverts.
d. Persons who do not exercise regularly.
e. Diabetics.

Q110. In considering an RTW plan for an employee with Long COVID Syndrome, which one of the following statements is the best fit?

a. The worker with long COVID should be allowed to be actively involved in (re)designing his/her work.
b. An RTW plan should have the agreement of the manager, human resource professional, the employee and the union representative.
c. Occupational health professionals can play an important role.
d. RTW is best dealt with on an individual basis.
e. An RTW plan could include the following: a phased return, flexible work, time off for rehabilitation and medical appointments, fatigue management strategies and adapting work tasks.

Fumes, Mists, Dusts and Gases

Q111. In metal fume fever, which one of the following statements is the best fit?

a. Tolerance does not develop over the working week.
b. Onset is typically immediate.
c. Risk is increased with increasing thickness of metal in cutting operations.
d. Is typically caused by exposure to cadmium fume.
e. Is gradually progressive.

Q112. In regard to the characteristics of inhalation fever, which one of the following statements is the best fit?

a. Tachyphylaxis occurs in the minority of cases.
b. Heavier exposure does not result in more severe attacks.
c. Sensitisation is common.
d. Teflon can cause polymer fume fever.
e. Onset is usually after three or four hours, and chest X-rays show typical inhalation fever appearance.

Q113. In coal worker's pneumoconiosis, which one of the following statements is the best fit?

a. Severity of the disease does not vary according to composition of the coal.
b. Simple coal worker's pneumoconiosis is associated with an increased risk of lung cancer.
c. Progressive massive fibrosis (PMF) is associated with melanoptysis.
d. Caplan syndrome typically occurs in association with ankylosing spondylitis.
e. PMF now very uncommon in US coal miners compared with the 1970s.

Q114. In regard to siderosis, which one of the following is correct?

a. Is due to exposure to tin ore.
b. Results in finding of 'black lung' at post-mortem.

c. Results from exposure to mixtures of silicates.
d. Typically associated with abnormal lung function.
e. Is also known as welder's disease.

Q115. In those exposed to wood dust, which one of the following is correct?

a. Softwood dust arises from deciduous trees.
b. Hardwood dust arises from coniferous trees.
c. Exposure is associated with excess squamous cell carcinoma of the nose and sinus cavity.
d. Is not associated with anosmia.
e. IARC (International Agency for Research on Cancer) Group 1 carcinogen.

Q116. In regard to ozone, which one of the following statements is correct?

a. In urban areas of dense population ozone tends to increase in inverse relationship to temperature.
b. It is better to use natural rubber seals and gaskets if the ozone concentration is likely to be increased.
c. The gas is readily detected by its chlorine-like smell at 0.1 ppm but is unlikely to cause respiratory problems until 5 ppm.
d. Ozone is not included in the CLP Regulation because it is always generated on site.
e. It is heavier than air so tends to rise inside buildings.

Q117. In regard to ozone gas, which one of the following is correct?

a. Is typically colourless.
b. Is pungent in low concentrations (less than 2 ppm).
c. Is a liquid or gas depending on temperature.
d. Produced in the breakdown of silage.
e. Is more soluble in water than in non-polar solvents.

Q118. Concerning carbon disulphide (CS2), which one of the following is correct?

a. Most absorbed CS2 is not metabolised and metabolites do not appear in the urine.
b. CS2 is a solvent used in MDF board manufacture.
c. Toxic effects include encephalopathy with mania and delusions.
d. Chronic exposure is associated with increased mortality from pancreatic disease.
e. Is an additive for oils and resins.

Q119. In regard to carbon monoxide, which one of the following is the best fit?

a. Carboxyhaemoglobin concentration is usually more than 10% in smokers.
b. Causes the oxyhemoglobin dissociation curve to shift to the right.
c. Is a by-product of the complete combustion of carbon fuels.
d. Occurs after exposure to methylene chloride.
e. There is no normal baseline human carboxyhemoglobin level.

Q120. Which one of the following gases is a chemical asphyxiant?

a. Nitrogen.
b. Methane.
c. Carbon dioxide.
d. Hydrogen sulphide.
e. Ammonia.

Q121. In regard to sulphur dioxide gas, which one of the following is correct?

a. Is the chemical compound with the formula SO.
b. Is insoluble in water.
c. Is yellow in colour.
d. Has no effect on pregnancy.
e. Particulate matter refers to the combined solid and liquid particles in air.

Q122. Which one of the following describes the property of hydrogen cyanide (HCn)?

a. Exposure results in a characteristic taste of garlic.
b. Interferes with anaerobic metabolism.
c. Has a brown colour at room temperature.
d. Thiocyanate levels accurately reflect intensity of intoxication.
e. Results in lactic acidosis.

Q123. Regarding carbon monoxide, which one of the following statements is the best fit?

a. Carbon monoxide exerts its toxic effect by binding to haemoglobin to produce carboxyhaemoglobin.
b. Chronic exposure to carbon monoxide accelerates atherogenesis.
c. Carbon monoxide contributes to the coronary and peripheral atherosclerosis experienced by cigarette smokers.
d. Haem containing proteins other than haemoglobin (e.g., myoglobin, cytochrome oxidase) also bind to carbon monoxide contributing further to its toxicity.
e. In maternal exposure, the concentration of blood carboxyhaemoglobin is greater than 10% higher than in the mother's blood.

General OH Practice and Legal Issues

Q124. Concerning aspects of confidentiality, which one of the following statements is incorrect?

a. General Data Protection Regulation indicates that consent is always required when processing a worker's information in occupational health settings.
b. Obtaining signed consent to provide a report prior to a telephone or video consultation with an employee is the best procedure.
c. If an employee decides to withhold a report from their employer, it should be deleted from their health record.
d. A method of confirming the employee's identity is advisable during a telephone consultation, also their location should be confirmed.
e. It is illegal for an employee to record a consultation without the consent of all parties.

Q125. The common law of tort has implications for the workplace because of which one of the following statements?

a. It defines the principles of civil litigation.
b. It forms the basis for Health and Safety Legislation.
c. It is a statutory instrument.
d. It governs employment law.
e. It relates to working hours.

Q126. For a civil claim to succeed all the following must exist with the exception of which one?

a. Duty of care.
b. Breach of the duty of care.
c. Breach of statutory duty.
d. Harm arises out of a breach of duty.
e. The loss was foreseeable.

Q127. All the following are potential reasons for a fair dismissal from work with the exception of which one?

a. Lack of capability.
b. Poor attendance.
c. Poor conduct.
d. Redundancy.
e. Lack of competence.

Q128. In regard to the importance of taking an occupational history, which one of the following does NOT fit?

a. Deals with the effect of work on health.
b. Hobbies and pastime activities should be included.
c. Previous jobs are as important as the current job.
d. Will always involve a detailed assessment of exposure to workplace hazards.
e. Allows an assessment to be made on fitness to return to work after illness or injury.

Q129. In regard to ill-health retirement, which one of the following does NOT fit?

a. It should be considered only when it is clear that an employee's health problem prevents a return to previous employment.
b. An employer cannot dismiss an employee with a genuine health problem.
c. The occupational physician may recommend it if the work environment would continually affect an employee's health adversely.
d. The company occupational physician is usually well placed to give advice.
e. It is the occupational physician's duty to ensure that redeployment has been considered before proceeding with the recommendation.

Q130. In regard to disabled workers, which one of the following is the best fit?

a. Have a higher than average rate of absence.
b. Restrictions (if any) should be appropriate and precise.
c. Only employed under employment disabled quota schemes.
d. Represent an increased safety risk in the workplace.
e. Will achieve limited benefit from the occupational health team.

Q131. When considering sickness absence, which one of the following is incorrect?

a. It is any absence from work attributed to incapacity.
b. Can be measured in a variety of ways, including percentage of time lost and average length of spells.
c. Young people tend to take more uncertified absence than the older worker.
d. Genuine medical illness exists in most cases.
e. Past attendance record is a good predictor of future attendance.

Q132. When considering the control of sickness absence, which one of the following statements does NOT fit?

a. Pre-employment medicals are good predictors.
b. Management has a responsibility for control.
c. A comprehensive written policy on sickness absence is useful in dealing with this issue.
d. Keeping staff informed on their levels of absence is worthwhile.
e. The International Labour Organization does not endorse an occupational physician being asked to justify or directly refute another physician's incapacity certificate.

Q133. In regard to alcohol problems in the workplace, which one of the following statements does NOT fit?

a. This may be indicated by a pattern of Monday absenteeism and deteriorating work performance.
b. The occupational health team should be involved in all aspects of a disciplinary policy, including taking samples of blood or urine.
c. An alcohol policy should be agreed by all, including top management.
d. Alcohol abuse in the workplace should, in the interests of the problem drinker, be treated in confidence.
e. The rules and penalties governing problem drinking must be clearly stated in an alcohol policy.

Q134. When considering workplace health promotion, which one of the following is the best fit?

a. It should form part of a comprehensive occupational health service.
b. A needs assessment is a useful first step.
c. It can link in with local and national health strategies.
d. Engaging with the workforce is beneficial to success.
e. Must have the support of management.

Q135. You have been asked to plan a well-being programme for your company. Which one of the following is the best fit?

a. Increase worker awareness of well-being needs.
b. Ensure workers understand what well-being offerings are available.
c. Take steps to overcome apathy and mistrust.
d. Keep participation time with reasonable timescales.
e. Worker engagement will benefit participation.

Q136. When compiling an effective occupational health (OH) report, which one of the following does NOT fit?

a. It must be in writing, using language that can be easily understood by a non-medical audience.
b. Be of practical value to personnel/management and the employee.
c. Should be focused and deal with matters of employment and fitness for work.
d. Contain relevant and appropriate medical information, including any interventions.
e. Allows HR/management to achieve a full understanding of the employee's situation.

Q137. You are asked to provide an OH report following assessment of a worker with multiple sclerosis. Which one of the following statements is the best fit?

a. It should advise whether the condition is likely to be covered by disability discrimination legislation and if adjustments to the job would be appropriate, and if these are likely to be temporary or permanent.
b. It should indicate if it appears that the employee's medical condition is related to their work, including any allegations of internal disputes that may require management assessment.
c. It should provide an opinion on the impact of the employee's health condition on future attendance or performance and whether retirement on health grounds may be appropriate.
d. It should indicate if a case conference with HR or management would be helpful, or if a workplace visit would provide further information that would assist in providing advice.
e. A report from the worker's general practitioner or hospital doctor may enable a better understanding of any underlying medical condition.

Q138. In regard to writing an OH report, which one of the following statements does NOT fit?

a. Reports should be clear, focused on the individual, relevant to their condition and job requirements and assist the manager/HR in the management of the case.
b. How information is obtained, for what purpose, and how it is stored is not an important consideration at the OH consultation.
c. Consent and how it is obtained are important considerations.
d. The role of OH within an organisation should be made available to all employees.
e. The employee being seen should understand why they are being assessed.

Q139. When carrying out an OH assessment leading to the preparation of a report, which one of the following is incorrect?

a. OH should ensure that the employee understands the reason for the referral prior to any assessment taking place.
b. What OH intends to do, including preparing a report and with whom this will be shared and why should be explained.
c. Having explained the issue of confidentiality, if this is a management referral, the assessment may continue without obtaining the express consent from the employee.
d. Consent to send a report to the manager should be obtained in writing from the employee.
e. In certain jurisdictions, the employee has the right to see a report before it is sent to management and certain time limits are usually applied.

Q140. When preparing an OH report for an employer, which one of the following types of employee information does NOT fit regarding sensitive personal data and the principles of data protection?

a. Staff number.
b. Date of birth.
c. Medical diagnosis.
d. Medication being taken.
e. Telephone number.

Q141. When considering what makes a good OH report, which one of the following statements is the best fit?

a. Never read out the referral to the employee if a box is ticked indicating the referral was discussed.
b. You do not need to consider changing an opinion in a report if the employee queries it.
c. Once the employee has signed the consent at the end of the consultation, they cannot change their mind.
d. Function details of the employee are not important in a report, just answer the questions.
e. Opinion given in an occupational health report is advice to the employer and they are free to ignore it if they chose.

Q142. When considering the provision of a OH report, which one of the following does NOT fit in regard to the worker's informed consent?

a. Provision of adequate information.
b. Provision of opportunity to discuss and consider the options.
c. Ensuring that the person has capacity to make the decision.
d. Obtaining the person's voluntary agreement.
e. Ensuring documentation is in writing.

Q143. Quality report writing is a key communication tool for occupational health (OH) practitioners and can be viewed as part of a reciprocal process, usually a response to a request from a line manager. Which one of the following statements is NOT a prerequisite to the provision of a quality report in this context?

a. An indication that the referring line manager has informed the employee about the process and obtained verbal consent to proceed.
b. The provision of demographic details and job title.
c. The principle of 'no surprises' for the employee when report is issued.
d. Informed consent prior to issuing a report to be obtained by the OH professional.
e. Reports should be accurate and attentive to detail as they may later become public.

Health Surveillance

Q144. In regard to health surveillance, which one of the following statements is incorrect?

a. Health surveillance is important for detecting ill-health effects at an early stage, so employers can introduce better controls to prevent them from getting worse.
b. Health surveillance can provide data to help employers evaluate health risks.
c. Health surveillance provides an opportunity to employees to raise concerns about how work affects their health.
d. Health surveillance is important for highlighting lapses in workplace control measures, therefore providing invaluable feedback to the risk assessment.
e. Health surveillance can be used as a substitute for undertaking a risk assessment or using effective controls.

Q145. Which one of the following is NOT an Occupational Health Surveillance Programme?

a. Hearing Conservation Programme.
b. Hand–Arm Vibration Surveillance.

c. Body Mass Index Measurement Programme.
d. Respiratory Protection Programme.
e. Skin Surveillance Programme.

Q146. Hierarchy of hazard control is a system used in industry to minimise or eliminate exposure to hazards. Which one of the following places a health surveillance programme in the context of the hierarchy of hazard control?

a. Elimination, substitution, engineering controls, administration controls, personal protective equipment, health surveillance.
b. Elimination, health surveillance, substitution, engineering controls, administration controls, personal protective equipment.
c. Elimination, substitution, health surveillance, engineering controls, administration controls, personal protective equipment.
d. Elimination, substitution, engineering controls, health surveillance, administration controls, personal protective equipment.
e. Elimination, substitution, engineering controls, administration controls, health surveillance, personal protective equipment.

Q147. Regarding health surveillance, which one of the following statements is the best fit?

a. Health surveillance should be supported by a policy approved by management and employees or their representatives.
b. Health surveillance programmes are necessary where workers are exposed to biological agents of Groups 3 and 4.
c. Test results obtained through health surveillance should be shared only with the individual employee participants.
d. A health surveillance programme for workers exposed to skin irritants (or sensitisers) should include an annual questionnaire.
e. Health surveillance programmes should include only those for whom baseline data from pre-employment health assessment is available.

Q148. Which one of the following is NOT a type of health surveillance?

a. Biological monitoring.
b. Self-reporting of symptoms.
c. Inspection by a responsible person who is not a nurse or a doctor.
d. Online questionnaire.
e. Blood tests.

Q149. Regarding health surveillance, which one of the following statements is the best fit?

a. Everyone who works with lead must have regular blood tests.
b. Blood tests are required for persons exposed to chemicals at work.
c. Night shift workers need to be physically examined once every year.
d. Only a risk assessment determines what is appropriate.
e. The Safety Data Sheet (SDS) determines what is appropriate.

Q150. Which one of the following is NOT a contraindication to performing spirometry?

a. Myocardial infarction (MI) in the previous four weeks.
b. Suspected aortic aneurism.
c. Cataract surgery seven days prior.
d. Haemoptysis of unknown origin.
e. Acute gastroenteritis.

Q151. In regard to audiometry, which one of the following is correct?

a. Is not required if adequate hearing protection is provided at work.
b. Can be done only in an audiometric booth.
c. Typically utilises a Hughson–Westlake method.
d. Distinguishes a conductive from a sensorineural loss.
e. Can diagnose acoustic neuromas.

In regard to definitions, match the following:

Q152. Illuminance.

Q153. Luminous intensity.

Q154. Luminance.

Q155. Reflectance.

Q156. Luminous flux.

a. Power of a source to emit light.
b. Luminous flux reflected: luminous flux incident.
c. The intensity of light falling on a surface.
d. The light emitted by a source or received by a surface.
e. The physical brightness of a surface.

Mental Health, Psychosocial Work Environment and Stress

Q157. Maslow's hierarchy of needs is a motivational theory in psychology comprising a five-tier model of human needs, often depicted as hierarchical levels within a pyramid. Needs lower down in the hierarchy must be satisfied before individuals can attend to needs higher up. From the bottom of the hierarchy upwards, which one of the following is correct?

a. Physiological, safety and security, love and belonging, self-esteem, self-actualisation.
b. Safety and security, physiological, love and belonging, self-actualisation, self-esteem.
c. Love and belonging, physiological, self-esteem, safety and security, self-actualisation.
d. Self-actualisation, physiological, safety and security, self-esteem, love and belonging.
e. Self-esteem, physiological, self-actualisation, love and belonging, safety and security.

Q158. Obesity is a chronic, relapsing, often disabling disease. Which one of the following statements is NOT true in regard to employees who are obese?

a. Increased sickness absence.
b. Decreased presenteeism.

c. Early retirement.
d. Ergonomic issues.
e. Work stress.

Q159. Well-being theory, as outlined by Martin Seligman, can be summarised in the PERMA model best described by which one of the following statements?

a. The model incorporates mindfulness and affect as individual elements.
b. The model incorporates physical fitness and engagement as individual elements.
c. The components are eudaimonic rather than hedonic.
d. Working on aspects of PERMA decreases psychological distress.
e. Each element is intrinsically motivating and contributes to well-being.

Q160. A meta-analysis for pharmacological treatment of post-traumatic stress disorder (PTSD) found evidence for which one of the following treatments?

a. Mirtazapine.
b. Fluoxetine.
c. Duloxetine.
d. Olanzapine.
e. Alprazolam.

Q161. Which one of the following interventions is NOT appropriate in the management of PTSD?

a. EMDR.
b. Cognitive processing therapy.
c. Watchful waiting if symptoms are mild for the first four weeks.
d. Psychological debriefing after traumatic event.
e. Prolonged exposure therapy.

Q162. In the UK Health and Safety Executive guidance, which one of the following is NOT one of the work areas recognised as a primary stress source?

a. Canteen food.
b. Change.
c. Control.
d. Support.
e. Role.

Q163. In considering personality disorder, which one of the following statements is correct?

a. Personality disorder is thought to be relatively common and easily diagnosed with the appropriate rating scale.
b. More than 50% of people with a personality disorder have a substance abuse problem, including alcohol.
c. People with personality disorders were felt to be untreatable but more recently there is evidence of successful approaches despite the high drop-out rates.
d. Personality disorders are innate traits and quite unlikely to come under the equality legislation.
e. The diagnostic criteria for obsessive-compulsive disorder are effectively the same as the obsessive-compulsive personality disorder but the treatment is different.

Q164. Burnout is reported as being common in certain service occupations. Which one of the following statements is the best fit?

a. Burnout is a clinical condition which overlaps in its presentation with depression.
b. Burnout is largely a euphemistic concept with no clear clinical basis.
c. Burnout is synonymous with emotional exhaustion.
d. Burnout is characterised by emotional exhaustion, reduced professional efficacy and increased mental distance from one's job.
e. Burnout is characterised by low mood and emotional exhaustion.

Q165. The UK's Health and Safety Executive's Management Standards framework for stress incorporates several work areas in which stress may be experienced. Which one of the following theories/models of stress is this approach based on?

a. The transactional model of stress.
b. The job demand–control–support model.
c. The person–environment fit.
d. The conservation of resources theory.
e. The effort–reward imbalance theory.

Q166. Job control is the extent to which individuals can influence their environment at work. It is measured in many of the widely used models of stress. Which one of the following statements is the best fit?

a. Job control is one element of the allostatic load model of stress.
b. Research has established a causal link between control (in various forms) at work and physical and psychological health.
c. Control is consistently shown as a buffer for the demands of work.
d. Studies on job control have had methodological issues which limit the degree to which one can infer a causal relationship between lack of control and work stress.
e. There is a strong relationship between perceived control and locus of control.

Q167. Organisational justice (OJ) is a model of occupational stress. Which one of the following statements is the best fit?

a. Procedural justice and relational justice are associated with negative mental health outcomes.
b. The OJ model is composed of procedural justice, relational justice and interactional justice.
c. The OJ model is composed of procedural, informational and distributive justice.
d. Procedural justice is the most frequently measured component of organisational justice.
e. The OJ model emphasises individual as well as interpersonal comparisons.

Q168. Which one of the following is NOT part of the UK Health and Safety Executive Management Standards for workplace stress?

a. Job demands.
b. Control over work.
c. Relationships at work.
d. Collective bargaining arrangements.
e. Supports at work.

Q169. Regarding the effort–reward imbalance (ERI) theoretical model of work stress, which one of the following statements is the best fit?

a. The model is firmly embedded in the person-environment (P-E) fit model of stress.

b. The model equally incorporates intrinsic and extrinsic components of stress.
c. The model's intrinsic component of over-commitment moderates effort and reward.
d. Over-commitment is causally linked to cardiovascular risk factors.
e. There is evidence of more adverse health impact from its extrinsic than intrinsic components.

Q170. Which one of the following statements is the best fit in relation to somatic symptom disorders (SSDs) or somatisation?

a. Cognitive behavioural therapy is the most effective therapeutic intervention in SSDs.
b. A strong doctor–patient relationship is key to making progress in SSDs.
c. It can occur when workers are faced with life changes (personal or occupational) and have inadequate coping skills.
d. Diagnosis requires persistent symptoms typically for at least six months *(DSM-5)*.
e. It complicates workplace injuries contributing to disability and delayed recovery.

Q171. Which one of the following is the best fit in regard to post-traumatic stress disorder (PTSD)?

a. Can occur after relatively trivial incidents in the workplace.
b. Can follow bullying in the workplace.
c. Can be diagnosed only after a perceived intense event associated with a threat to life.
d. Is underdiagnosed in cases of litigation.
e. Becomes more likely when an event is recurrent.

Q172. In dealing with COVID-19, which one of the following key elements does NOT fit when protecting the mental health of healthcare workers (HCWs)?

a. Early support of HCWs for the situation and dilemmas they will face.
b. Ongoing monitoring by supportive team leaders.
c. Access to peer support programmes, psychological therapies and mental health support.
d. Staff who do not turn up to work should not be contacted at home.
e. As normality returns all HCWs should receive 'return to normal work' interviews.

Musculoskeletal Disorders and Ergonomics

Q173. Frozen shoulder typically resolves in which one of the following timescales?

a. One week.
b. Three weeks.
c. Six weeks.
d. Three months.
e. Eighteen months.

Q174. A red flag in low back pain is which one of the following?

a. Fear of re-injury.
b. Low job satisfaction.
c. Gait disturbance.
d. Fear of movement.
e. Use of regular analgesics.

Q175. A yellow flag in low back pain is which one of the following?

a. Fear avoidance behaviour.
b. Weight loss.
c. Litigation.
d. Poor job satisfaction.
e. Unrelenting nausea.

Q176. A 42-year-old woman working as an operative in a textile factory presents with intermittent ill-defined pain in her right forearm and paraesthesia of all fingers. She presents as somewhat anxious and clinical examination of her forearm is normal. You make a provisional diagnosis of work-related upper limb disorder (WRULD). Which one of the following options is least likely to be helpful in the initial management of her case?

a. Referral for electrophysiological studies.
b. An exploration of psychosocial risk factors.
c. Examination of her cervical spine.
d. An ergonomic assessment of her workstation.
e. Temporary work restrictions and early review.

Q177. Which one of the following clinical tests of the upper limb is useful in clinical practice?

a. The 'scarf test' is used to test the integrity of the sternoclavicular joint.
b. The 'empty can' test is useful for assessing the function of the infraspinatus muscle.
c. Phalen's manoeuvre is moderately accurate in mimicking symptoms of radial tunnel syndrome.
d. Finkelstein's test is helpful in confirming the diagnosis of de Quervain's tenosynovitis.
e. Gerber's lift-off test is accurate in assessing the function of the supraspinatus muscle.

Q178. Characteristic features of carpal tunnel syndrome are which one of the following?

a. Ulnar nerve distribution of tingling and pain.
b. Pain or numbness worse during daytime.
c. Pains in the wrist radiating into the forearm.
d. Median nerve distribution of absence of sensation.
e. Positive Mill's test.

Q179. In lateral epicondylitis (tennis elbow) the tendinous origin of which one of the following muscles is most often involved?

a. Extensor carpi radialis brevis.
b. Extensor carpi ulnaris.
c. Extensor digitorum.
d. Extensor digiti minimi.
e. Extensor carpi radialis longus.

Q180. Considering lateral epicondylitis, which one of the following is the best fit?

a. Affects 5% of adults annually.
b. Both arms are equally affected.

c. Most common between ages of 35 and 50.
d. Men are more frequently affected.
e. Requires an MRI scan to confirm diagnosis.

Q181. In regard to Dupuytren's disease (DD), which one of the following statements is NOT true?

a. DD has a significant genetic involvement.
b. DD is associated with high alcohol consumption.
c. DD is not associated with smoking.
d. DD is associated with diabetes.
e. DD is associated with carpal tunnel syndrome.

Q182. Carpal tunnel syndrome (CTS) is recognised as being associated with which one of the following?

a. Exposure to vibrating hand tools.
b. Prolonged keyboard work with normal posture.
c. Pregnancy.
d. Genetic factors account for most cases.
e. Ulnar nerve is affected.

Q183. Which one of the following is a 'blue flag' in terms of back pain?

a. Belief that work is too onerous and likely to cause further injury.
b. Legislation restricting options for return to work.
c. Conflict with insurance staff over injury claim.
d. Overly concerned family and healthcare providers.
e. Heavy work, with little opportunity to modify duties.

Q184. When examining a patient with potential carpal tunnel syndrome, which one of the following is the most sensitive clinical sign?

a. Tinel's sign.
b. Phalen's sign.
c. Square wrist sign.
d. Carpal compression test.
e. Finkelstein's sign.

Q185. In regard to carpal tunnel syndrome (CTS), which one of the following statements does NOT fit?

a. CTS is widely accepted as being the most common peripheral nerve entrapment syndrome, with a 10% lifetime risk of the condition.
b. The median nerve entrapment occurs as it passes through the carpal tunnel on the palmar aspect of the wrist.
c. The sensory symptoms of CTS reflect the sensory distribution of that nerve, being the thumb, index and middle fingers and the lateral aspect of the ring finger, and the corresponding area of the palm.
d. Sensory symptoms involving the little finger never occur in CTS.
e. A differential diagnosis includes sensorineural hand–arm vibration syndrome (HAVS).

Q186. The level of evidence for a range of workstation interventions to reduce the prevalence of upper extremity musculoskeletal disorders (UEMSDs) varies from strong to insufficient. Which one of the following statements is the best fit?

a. There is moderate evidence to support the recommendation of alternative/split keyboards.
b. There is moderate evidence to support the recommendation of tracker ball devices.
c. There is moderate evidence to support the use of forearm supports.
d. There is no evidence to support the use of a tactile feedback signal on computer mouse.
e. There is moderate evidence to support the recommendation of a joystick pointing device.

Q187. A 32-year-old office worker complains of increasing pain in her neck and shoulders later in the working day, getting worse as the week progresses and better at the weekend. Which one of the following ergonomic alterations is most likely to improve her symptoms?

a. Lower her chair height.
b. Ensure support for upper back while seated.
c. Raise screen.
d. Ensure lumbar lordosis is maintained.
e. Raise the chair height.

Q188. In considering the compilation of an ergonomic programme within a telephone call centre, which one of the following statements is the best fit?

a. Surveillance of health and safety records including sickness absence data to determine any patterns of MSDs.
b. Carry out a job analysis to find out ergonomic hazards present and worker exposure to these.
c. Consider as necessary job redesign to eliminate or reduce ergonomic hazards.
d. Training employers and employee in the identification of ergonomic hazards.
e. Carry out annual upper limb and neck surveillance.

Q189. When working at a seated workstation, which one of the following statements is correct?

a. Bifocal lenses should be removed.
b. Screen height should be higher if using bifocal lenses.
c. Screen height should be between 0 and 30 degrees above eye level for most users.
d. Screen height should be lower for users of bifocal lenses.
e. The most important determinant of head posture is the height of the work surface.

Noise, Vibration and Thermal Environment

Q190. A worker is exposed to 72 dB Leq for four hours. He is then exposed to 82 dB Leq for three hours and 92 dB Leq for one hour. His overall noise exposure for the eight hours Leq is approximately which one of the following?

a. 75 dB.
b. 78 dB.
c. 81 dB.
d. 84 dB.
e. 88 dB.

Q191. For hearing protection for noise exposure, which one of the following is the best fit?

a. Is compulsory once the A8 exposure exceeds 80 dB.
b. Is always an early consideration in management of significant noise exposure.
c. Needs to be worn at least 85% of the time the employee is exposed to significant noise to be effective.
d. Should be worn in a designated hearing protection zone even if the noise level is between the upper and lower action levels.
e. Is more likely to be required in confined spaces.

Q192. In regard to noise assessment and noise-induced hearing loss (NIHL), which one of the following statements is the best fit?

a. Raising the noise level by 5 dB has the effect of doubling sound levels.
b. Reduced hearing of consonants is often the first impairment in speech interpretation noticed in NIHL which is typical in the higher frequency end of the speech band.
c. The A-weighting scale mirrors the response of the human ear at different frequencies to create an equivalent loudness at 50 dB.
d. The typical 4 kHz notch in NIHL is primarily due to the shape of the cochlea and poor blood supply in the first bend in the cochlea where the 4 kHz region is located.
e. Prior to audiometry the worker should not have been exposed to excess noise for 48 hours.

Q193. In regard to age-related hearing loss, which one of the following is the best fit?

a. Must be distinguished from presbycusis.
b. Results in rapid deterioration of hearing.
c. Has a genetic component in 50% of cases.
d. Is associated with a notch on the audiogram.
e. Affects the lower frequencies first.

Q194. In regard to A- and C-weighting of sound pressure levels, which one of the following is the best fit?

a. Are used because the human ear is more sensitive to certain frequencies than to others.
b. A-weighting should be applied when measuring peak sound pressure.
c. C-weighting mimics the response of the human ear.
d. Are measured in the performance of audiometry.
e. In A-weighting the decibel values of sounds at low frequencies are increased, compared with unweighted decibels.

In regard to noise, match the following:

Q195. dB(A).

Q196. Lep'd.

Q197. Second action level.

Q198. Noise dose.

Q199. Peak action level.

a. Depends on level of noise and exposure time.
b. 140 dB.
c. Noise weighting that closely simulates the human ear.
d. Level of daily continual personal exposure.
e. Hearing protection mandatory.

Q200. In relation to hand–arm vibration syndrome (HAVS), which one of the following is the best fit?

a. Is categorised using the Griffin score.
b. Workers exposed to tools with a dominant frequency in the range of 60–300 Hz are more likely to develop the symptoms of HAVS.
c. Workers using hand tools that emit a lower dominant frequency (i.e., 10–60 Hz) are more likely to have neurological symptoms.
d. Is typically wholly symmetrical.
e. Rarely improves after removal from vibration.

Q201. Long-term, regular exposure to hand–arm vibration (HAV) is known to lead to potentially permanent and debilitating health effects known as hand–arm vibration syndrome, vibration white finger and carpal tunnel syndrome. Which one of the following clinical tests is not useful in a HAVS clinical assessment?

a. Allen's test.
b. Jobe's test.
c. Phalen's manouevre.
d. Roos stress test.
e. Finkelstein's test.

Q202. A male employee has tingling in the index, middle and ring fingers of his left hand that lasts for 10 minutes after he stops using his angle grinder. Which one of the following statements is the best fit?

a. The tingling is likely to be due to hand–arm vibration syndrome (HAVS).
b. Further assessment is required, including an assessment of temperature and vibration thresholds.
c. The diagnosis is unlikely to be carpal tunnel syndrome (CTS) because the thumb is not involved.
d. Usually tingling or numbness that has a duration of 20 minutes or more is regarded as likely to be significant in relation to hand-transmitted vibration.
e. A smoking history is not relevant.

Q203. When considering whole-body vibration (WBV) exposure, which one of the following is the best fit?

a. Not affected by road surface.
b. Not affected by road speed.
c. Not affected by vehicle suspension.
d. Not affected by cold environment.
e. WBV typically results in decreased bone mass.

Q204. Based on the Stockholm Workshop Scale for classification of vibration white finger stage 2, which one of the following is the best fit?

a. No attacks.
b. Occasional attacks affecting the distal and middle phalanges of one or more fingers.
c. Occasional attacks affecting the tips of one or more fingers.
d. Trophic skin changes in the fingertips.
e. Objective evidence of vascular obstruction is required.

Q205. In regard to whole-body vibration, which one of the following statements is the best fit?

a. High intensity exposure is typically better tolerated for longer periods then low intensity exposure.
b. Visual performance is impaired in the range of 1,000 Hz.
c. Horizontal vibration is more harmful than vertical vibration for seated workers.
d. Effect does not depend on frequency of vibration.
e. Stiff seats may amplify the effect of vibration.

Q206. Exposure to whole-body vibration (WBV) occurs in many occupations, including mining, farming and heavy equipment operators. Based on a high level of evidence (e.g., systematic review), which one of the following statements is the best fit?

a. In farmers there is a strong causal link between exposure to WBV and low back pain.
b. Workers exposed to WBV are at significantly greater risk of being hospitalised due to lumbar disc herniation.
c. Workers exposed to WBV are at significantly greater risk of low back pain and sciatica.
d. Male workers exposed to WBV have a significantly increased risk of prostate cancer.
e. WBV as a therapeutic intervention improves bone mass in older women.

Q207. In relation to whole-body vibration and health effects, which one of the following is the best fit?

a. Lumbar disc degeneration.
b. Menstrual disorders.
c. Autonomic disorders.
d. Sciatica.
e. Simple low back pain.

Q208. Slaughterhouses and meat packing plants are conducive to SARS-CoV-2 transmission. Which one of the following is NOT widely associated with SARS-CoV-2-transmission in such workplaces?

a. Low temperatures.
b. Air recirculation.
c. Non-metal surfaces.
d. Aerosolisation aggravated by high-volume water use.
e. Hyperpnoea because of heavy manual labour.

Q209. When considering Wet Bulb Globe Temperature (WBGT), which one of the following is the best fit?

a. Is a measure of heat stress in the shade.
b. Considers ambient temperature and humidity only.
c. Wind speed is not a factor.
d. Sun angle is a factor.
e. Is no longer regularly used as a measurement.

Q210. In regard to heat exhaustion, which one of the following does not fit?

a. Confusion.
b. Loss of appetite.
c. Tachycardia.
d. Failure to sweat.
e. Temperature at 38°C or above.

Q211. Which one of the following is NOT a factor that can contribute to heat stroke?

a. Dehydration from not drinking enough water.
b. Being overweight.
c. Sleep deprivation, which can decrease the rate of sweating.
d. Taking an SSRI.
e. Being unaccustomed to the heat.

Q212. All of the following are symptoms of hypothermia with the exception of which one?

a. Shivering.
b. Failure to shiver.
c. Pinpoint pupils.
d. Confusion.
e. Loss of consciousness.

Q213. In regard to heat stroke, which one of the following statements does NOT fit?

a. Heat stroke is a medical emergency with a high mortality if not diagnosed and treated appropriately.
b. The core body temperature of a patient with heat stroke is no greater than 39°C.
c. Heat stroke is due to a failure in the thermoregulatory mechanism.
d. There may be tissue damage to the liver, kidneys and brain in the absence of sweating.
e. Rapid cooling is required by wetting and measures to increase evaporation along with supportive measures such as an intravenous infusion.

Q214. In regard to hypothermia, which one of the following statements does NOT fit?

a. Hypothermia is diagnosed when the core temperature is less than 35°C.
b. The absence of shivering is a good prognostic indicator.
c. The hypothermic patient may experience delirium, coma and death.
d. First aid management includes the application of thermal blankets.
e. Hypothermia may be complicated with an acid base imbalance.

Match the following thermal components with one from the following list:

Q215. Convection.

Q216. Thermoregulatory mechanisms.

Q217. Radiation.

Q218. Evaporation.

Q219. Effective temperature index.

a. Does not depend on air movement.
b. A measure of temperature, humidity and air velocity.
c. Dependent on air temperature and velocity.
d. Peripheral vasodilatation and sweating.
e. Dependent on temperature, humidity and air velocity.

Occupational Cancer

Q220. Which one of the following compounds has NOT been designated a Group 1 human carcinogen by IARC (International Agency for Research on Cancer)?

a. Ethyl alcohol.
b. Formaldehyde.
c. Ethylene oxide.
d. Carbon tetrachloride.
e. Polychlorinated biphenyls (PCB).

Q221. Which one of the following is NOT classified by IARC as human carcinogens?

a. Aluminium production.
b. Acheson process to manufacture silicon carbide or graphite.
c. Strong inorganic mists.
d. Petrol engine exhaust.
e. Diesel engine exhaust.

Q222. In occupational cancer, which one of the following statements is correct?

a. Occupational cancer is the biggest cause of work-related death worldwide.
b. Around 4.5% of female breast cancer has been attributed to the IARC Group 1 classified shift work.
c. Asbestos is a significant cause of bladder cancer.
d. Radon is not a cause of occupational cancer.
e. Welding is a significant cause of liver angiosarcoma.

Q223. Which one of the following has been linked to the causation of angiosarcoma of the liver?

a. PVC.
b. Styrene monomer.
c. Mercury.
d. Arsenic containing insecticide.
e. Alcohol.

Q224. Which one of the following is not a risk factor for occupational cancer?

a. Hepatitis B virus infection.
b. Hepatitis C virus infection.
c. COVID-19 infection.
d. Exposure to tetrachlorethylene.
e. Work as a welder.

Q225. Screening for lung cancer is an example of which one of the following?

a. Primary prevention.
b. Secondary prevention.
c. Tertiary prevention.
d. All of the above.
e. None of the above.

Q226. Which one of the following types of leukaemia is most linked to occupational exposure?

a. Acute lymphoblastic leukaemia and acute myeloid leukaemia.
b. Acute lymphoblastic leukaemia and chronic lymphocytic leukaemia.
c. Acute myeloid leukaemia and chronic myeloid leukaemia.
d. Acute myeloid leukaemia and multiple myeloma.
e. Chronic myeloid leukaemia and chronic lymphocytic leukaemia.

Q227. Which one of the following is NOT a Group 1 carcinogen designated by IARC?

a. Aluminium production.
b. Alcohol.
c. Benzidine.
d. Night shift work.
e. Benzene.

In regard to these conditions, match the following:

Q228. Cancer of the skin.

Q229. Carcinoma of the bladder.

Q230. Tumour of the liver.

Q231. Bronchial carcinoma.

Q232. Nasal cancer.

a. Aromatic amines.
b. Vinyl chloride monomer (VCM).
c. Pitch, cutting oils and ultraviolet light.
d. Leather workers, hardwoods and nickel.
e. Uranium, nickel carbonyl, chromates and asbestos.

Occupational Hygiene

Q233. In occupational hygiene, which one of the following is the best fit for the Ames test?

a. Is primarily a test for carcinogenesis.
b. Is an in-vivo test.
c. Use an auxotrophic strain of bacteria.
d. Utilises Salmonella typhi bacteria.
e. Utilises a histidine-rich agar for culture.

Q234. In local exhaust ventilation, the term 'capture velocity' is defined by which one of the following?

a. The air velocity at the opening of a hood.
b. The minimum velocity required to keep collected particles airborne in a system.
c. The sum of the static and velocity pressures at a point in an airstream.
d. The air velocity required at the source of emission sufficient to cause the pollutant to move towards the mouth of the extractor.
e. Quantified by using a smoke test.

Q235. Dermal uptake of a chemical is determined by which one of the following?

a. Permeability coefficient of skin exposed.
b. Concentration of substance in the air.
c. Breathing rate.
d. Site of exposure.
e. Presence of hair.

Q236. In regard to health surveillance, which one of the following is correct?

a. Is the same as medical screening in the workplace.
b. Helps to distinguish between health effects from exposure and those from pre-existing medical conditions.
c. Is not required when exposures are below occupational exposure limits.
d. Is always required when there is exposure to asthma-causing agents.
e. Depends on the level of residual risk.

Q237. In relation to fumes, which one of the following statements is the best fit?

a. Benzene emits fumes at room temperature if not enclosed.
b. Carbon monoxide fumes can be measured with a direct reading instrument.
c. Fumes are typically less than 1 nm (nanometre) in diameter.
d. Are formed by evaporation from melting metal.
e. Fumes persist for hours after formation.

Q238. In ventilation, which one of the following best describes the term 'stack effect'?

a. Natural movements of air in a building created by wind flow.
b. Air movements attributable to chimneys or stacks.
c. Dispersion of emissions from chimneys.
d. Air movements created as warm air rises in a building.
e. Forced ventilation using axial fans in a stack.

Q239. Personal sampling pumps used for measurements in the workplace have variable flow rates. A standard flow pump has a flow rate of which one of the following?

a. 1–10 ml per minute.
b. 10–100 ml per minute.
c. 0.5–3 litres per minute.
d. 3–30 litres per minute.
e. 30–300 litres per minute.

Q240. The SI unit for luminous flux is which one of the following?

a. Lumen.
b. Candela.
c. Lux.
d. Luminosity.
e. All of the above.

In regard to aspects of occupational hygiene, match the following:

Q241. Occupational hygiene.

Q242. Hazard.

Q243. Risk.

Q244. OES: occupational exposure standard.

Q245. OEL: occupational exposure limit.

a. Substance with potential to cause harm.
b. Relate to adequate control of substances for COSHH.
c. Level to which employees can be exposed without harming their health.
d. Likelihood of harm occurring in conditions of use of a substance.
e. Science and practice of protecting health of persons at work by controlling their exposure to workplace hazards.

Match what the following are used to measure:

Q246. Draeger tube.

Q247. Kata thermometer.

Q248. Whirling hygrometer.

Q249. Pump-operated personal sampler.

Q250. Globe thermometer.

a. Air humidity.
b. Sampling of gases, vapours and dusts.
c. Radiant temperature.
d. Location sampling of gases and vapours.
e. Air velocity.

Match the following to their units of measurement:

Q251. Noise.

Q252. Airborne concentration of dusts.

Q253. Vapour concentration in air.

Q254. Asbestos dust.

Q255. Ionising radiation.

a. mg/m^3.
b. ppm.
c. dB.
d. Sievert.
e. Fibres/ml.

Q256. An employee works with both toluene and xylene. Both are measured in an occupational hygiene assessment. The results are that toluene levels are 50% of the occupational exposure limit (OEL) eight-hour time-weighted assessment. Similarly, xylene is measured at 60% of its OEL. Which one of the following is the best fit?

a. Control is satisfactory but ongoing monitoring is required.
b. Biological monitoring for xylene is indicated.
c. Biological monitoring for both toluene and xylene is indicated.
d. Control is unsatisfactory and immediate action is required.
e. Control is satisfactory and no further action is required.

Q257. In asbestos exposure, which one of the following is correct?

a. Most commonly occurs in quarries and mines.
b. Is associated with an excess of tuberculosis.
c. Asbestos is a class 1A carcinogen.
d. Has an additive effect with smoking.
e. Crocidolite is an example of serpentine asbestos.

Q258. Which one of the following is the best fit when considering PM1 (Particulate matter less than 1 μm)?

a. Is synonymous with nanoparticles.
b. Is a major component of construction dust emissions.
c. Is linked with respiratory mortality but not cardiovascular mortality.
d. Has a WHO Air Quality Guideline (AQG) established.
e. Has been linked with higher mortality in diabetics.

Q259. Which one of the following is NOT associated with exposure to asbestos?

a. Diffuse pleural thickening.
b. Pericarditis.
c. Chronic obstructive bronchitis.
d. Cancer of the larynx.
e. Pulmonary alveolar proteinosis (PAP).

Q260. Regarding nanomaterials, which one of the following statements is the best fit?

a. REACH defines nanomaterials in the range of 10 nm to 100 nm.
b. An aspect ratio of 1:6 defines fibrous nanomaterials.
c. Graphene-based carbon single-walled nanotubes are limited to an aspect ratio of 1:4 and therefore are viewed unlikely to cause respiratory disease.
d. In the absence of defined airborne exposure limits risk assessment for exposure to workers remains the primary procedure in industry.
e. A problem with nanomaterials and their potential health effects is that despite their size they are insoluble.

Radiation: Ionising and Non-Ionising

Q261. In regard to the ionising radiation dose limits for classified workers in the EU, which one of the following parameters apply per annum?

a. Not greater than 20 mSv overall and 15 mSv for the lens of the eye and 150 mSv for skin and extremities.
b. Not greater than 1 mSv overall and 5 mSv for the lens of the eye and 15 mSv for skin and extremities.
c. Not greater than 20 mSv overall and 20 mSv for the lens of the eye and 500 mSv for skin and extremities.
d. Not greater than 6 mSv overall and 15 mSv for the lens of the eye and 150 mSv for skin and extremities.
e. Not greater than 6 mSv overall and 15 mSv for the lens of the eye and 150 mSv for skin and extremities.

Q262. The adverse health effects of radiation exposure may be stochastic or deterministic. Which one of the following statements best fits this classification?

a. Radiation thyroiditis is a stochastic effect.
b. Heritable disorders are a stochastic effect.
c. Stochastic effects may also be called tissue reaction.
d. Radiation-induced lung injury is a stochastic effect.
e. Cancer induction is a deterministic effect.

Q263. Occupational doses of radiation in interventional procedures guided by fluoroscopy are the highest doses registered among medical staff using X-rays. Which one of the following statements is incorrect?

a. Ionising radiation accounts for risk-dose-dependent stochastic effects (no threshold dose).
b. Ionising radiation accounts for risk-dose-dependent deterministic effects (threshold dose).
c. Deterministic effects such as erythema or cataract have a threshold dose below which the biological response is not observed.
d. Stochastic effects such as induction of cancer and genetic defects are probabilistic events and are similar among individuals.
e. Chromosomal aberrations are the most fully developed biological indicator of ionising radiation exposure.

Q264. In regard to radon, which one of the following is the best fit?

a. Typically, in the UK, Scotland has the highest areas affected by radon gas production.
b. Radon is primarily a domestic housing issue and rarely relevant to workplaces.
c. Radon exposure increases the risk of liver and colon cancer though to a lesser extent than lung cancer.
d. Workplaces below ground are required under legislation to include the potential for radon exposure in their risk assessment.
e. Has a very pungent odour.

Q265. On average, a person receives 546 μSv per year from medical procedures. Which one of the following procedures gives rise to the highest exposure to radiation?

a. Mammography to identify breast cancer.
b. Dental X-ray.
c. Angiocardiogram to determine heart function.
d. CT scan.
e. Chest X-ray.

Q266. Which one of the following types of natural radiation contributes most to the exposure of the population in Ireland to natural radiation?

a. Cosmic radiation.
b. Natural radioactivity in soils.
c. Thoron.
d. Natural radioactivity in food.
e. Radon.

Q267. Health effects from radiation doses can be grouped into two categories: deterministic and stochastic. Which one of the following statements is incorrect in regard to deterministic effects?

a. Deterministic effects occur after a threshold dose is reached.
b. Deterministic effects occur by statistical chance.
c. Ionising radiation doses below the threshold are not expected to cause the effect.
d. The severity of the deterministic effect increases with the dose.
e. Skin reddening (erythema) is an example of a deterministic effect with a threshold dose of approximately 300 rad (3 Gy).

Q268. Health effects from radiation doses can be grouped into two categories: deterministic and stochastic. Which one of the following statements is incorrect in regard to stochastic effects?

a. Stochastic effects occur by statistical chance.
b. The probability of the effect occurring in a population increases with the dose received, and the severity of the effect does not depend on the dose.
c. Cancer is the main stochastic effect that can result from radiation dose, often many years following the exposure.
d. Stochastic health effects are assumed to have a threshold dose below which they do not occur.
e. Although it may not accurately describe all stochastic health effects, they are sometimes described as 'long-term' health effects.

Q269. Which one of the following types of ionising radiation can make objects radioactive?

a. Alpha particles.
b. Beta particles.
c. Neutron particles.
d. Gamma rays.
e. X-rays.

Q270. Which one of the following types of radiation has the least penetrating power?

a. Alpha particles.
b. Beta particles.
c. Neutron particles.
d. Gamma rays.
e. X-rays.

Q271. Which one of the following types of radiation has the most penetrating power?

a. Alpha particles.
b. Beta particles.
c. Neutron particles.
d. Gamma rays.
e. X-rays.

Q272. In regard to ionising radiation (IR) dose limits, which one of the following is correct?

a. Are different for classified and non-classified radiation workers.
b. Are recommended by the Atomic Energy Authority.
c Aim to prevent stochastic effects.
d. Aim to limit non-stochastic effects.
e. Controlled area is one which cannot be entered by classified persons.

Q273. When considering ionising radiation and personal monitoring, which one of the following statements is correct?

a. Film badges are less sensitive to low doses than thermoluminescent dosimeters (TLDs).
b. TLDs can be stored to provide a permanent record.
c. Film badges are less sensitive to heat and humidity.
d. Film badge information is destroyed on reading.
e. The risk assessment that will be required to keep doses as low as reasonably practicable does not include any use of personal protective equipment.

In regard to the following, match the correct response:

Q274. Beta particles.

Q275. Radioactivity.

Q276. Ionisation.

Q277. Gamma rays.

Q278. Alpha particles.

a. Cannot penetrate skin.
b. Very penetrative and very hazardous.
c. Spontaneous process of decay.
d. Radiations which release electrically charged particles in tissues.
e. Can penetrate skin to 1 cm and are hazardous to superficial tissues.

Q279. Non-ionising radiation includes all radiations and fields of the electromagnetic spectrum that do not normally have sufficient energy to produce ionisation in matter. As such it does not break bonds that hold molecules in cells together. Which one of the following types of radiation is NOT a type of non-ionising radiation?

a. Infrared.
b. Beta particles.
c. Extremely low frequency.
d. Lasers.
e. Ultraviolet.

Q280. In regard to luminance, which one of the following is correct?

a. Is measured in candela.
b. Units are lumens per square metre.
c. Is the term applied to luminous flux emitted per solid angle.
d. Is the flow of light in a given direction from a surface element.
e. Is the same as brightness.

Q281. Occupational photokeratitis typically results in which one of the following?

a. From exposure to visible light.
b. From exposure to infrared light.
c. From exposure to ultraviolet (UV) light.
d. In damage to the retina.
e. Damage is usually permanent.

Q282. Regarding radio frequency (RF), which one of the following statements is the best fit?

a. RF in high doses may cause heat and molecular ionisation.
b. RF is measured in volts per metre.
c. Extremely low frequency (ELF) radiation causes teratogenesis in the offspring of exposed males.
d. ELF radiation causes childhood leukaemia.
e. Thermal injury to workers from RF may be affected by environmental humidity.

Q283. Exposure to radio frequency electromagnetic fields (RF: EMF) can have adverse biological effects. Regarding the health effects of cell or mobile phones, which one of the following statements is the best fit?

a. Mobile phones and/or tablets emit radiofrequency waves below the microwave range.
b. Radio frequency electromagnetic fields have deleterious effects on sperm function.
c. Oxidative stress due to the production of reactive oxygen species (ROS) damage sperm parameters (e.g., count, morphology, motility).
d. Epidemiologic studies have found increased rates of acoustic neuroma.
e. Epidemiologic studies have found increased rates of brain tumours.

Q284. Non-ionising radiation incorporates a range of radio frequencies, including which one of the following?

a. Gamma rays, ultraviolet and infrared.
b. Infrared, visible and ultraviolet.
c. Alpha particles, infrared and ultraviolet.
d. Gamma rays, microwaves and ultraviolet.
e. Alpha particles, microwaves and visible.

Q285. Visible radiation (VR) can present as an occupational hazard in varied settings. Which one of the following statements is the best fit?

a. The lens is the part of the eye most sensitive to VR.
b. Insufficient lighting or reflected light (glare) can cause eye strain (asthenopia) with repeated episodes leading to ocular damage.
c. Blue light causes a destructive photochemical reaction responsible for solar retinitis.
d. Intense light sources (e.g., laser) cause thermal retinal damage.
e. Cataracts increase the risk of retinal damage by VR.

Q286. Regarding arc eye (photokeratitis), which one of the following is correct?

a. It is typically caused by exposure to UVA.
b. Onset of symptoms is typically six to eight hours after exposure.
c. The presence of associated lid chemosis is rare.
d. Fluorescein staining is usually negative due to oedema.
e. Can occur from exposure to infrared light.

Q287. In regard to lasers, which one of the following statements is the best fit?

a. Class 2 lasers can cause instantaneous retinal damage.
b. Class 4 lasers have such low energy that the risk of harm is minimal.
c. Class 1 lasers are rarely used because of health risks.
d. Class 3R lasers will cause retinal damage even on reflection.
e. Class 3B lasers have up to 100 times more energy than Class 3R lasers.

Q288. In regard to infrared light, which one of the following is correct?

a. Causes lens damage and affects the cornea.
b. Does not affect the retina.
c. Causes pain in the eye on exposure.
d. Personal protective equipment is of little use as the effect is primarily heating.
e. Is ionising radiation (IR).

Q289. Regarding electromagnetic fields (EMFs), which one of the following statements is the best fit?

a. An electric field increases as current increases.
b. Electric fields are measured in volts per square metre v/m^2.
c. A magnetic field increases as the current increases.
d. Electric fields are present only when a device is turned on.
e. Electric fields easily permeate walls.

Q290. Which one of the following sources of electromagnetic fields (EMFs) may present a risk to workers if the safe limits are exceeded?

a. Electrolysis as part of a manufacturing process.
b. Use of dielectric heating equipment.
c. Use of induction heating equipment.
d. Use of manually operated resistance welding equipment.
e. All of the above.

Respiratory Disorders

Q291. Serial peak flow recording for occupational asthma should take place over a period of at least which one of the following?

a. One week.
b. Two weeks.
c. Four weeks.
d. Six weeks.
e. Twelve weeks.

Q292. The diagnostic features of occupational asthma on a serial peak flow record are variable airflow obstruction with which one of the following?

a. Greater than 10% variation in peak flow values.
b. Greater than 20% variation in peak flow values.
c. Greater than 50% variation in peak flow values.
d. Greater than 80% variation in peak flow values.
e. Greater than 90% variation in peak flow values.

Q293. Aspergillus fumigatus has which one of the following properties?

a. Is a mould.
b. Is rapidly killed at temperatures above 45°C.
c. Does not cause an aspergilloma in an immunocompetent host.
d. Is rare in nature.
e. Allergic bronchopulmonary aspergillosis can be treated with oral corticosteroids.

Q294. A worker in a kitchen manufacturing company is incidentally found to have upper zone and mid-zone nodules on chest X-ray. Which one of the following is the most likely diagnosis?

a. Silicosis.
b. Asbestosis.
c. Chronic obstructive pulmonary disease (COPD).
d. Asthma.
e. Previous tuberculosis.

Q295. A heating company executive is referred with persistent breathlessness. He is a lifelong smoker. His general practitioner has organised a chest X-ray, which has been reported as showing bilateral pleural plaques as well hyperinflated lungs. On examination he has mild wheeze only. The most likely cause of his breathlessness is which one of the following?

a. Asbestosis.
b. Chronic obstructive pulmonary disease (COPD).
c. Idiopathic pulmonary fibrosis (IPF).
d. Mesothelioma.
e. Silicosis.

Q296. A PhD science student is referred with nasal symptoms. She works in a lab where trial drugs are tested on guinea pigs. From the history, she also describes some eye symptoms that started before nasal symptoms. The most likely immunological aetiology of her symptoms is which one of the following?

a. Contact dermatitis.
b. Respiratory sensitisation.
c. Exposure to irritant substances.
d. Hypersensitivity pneumonitis.
e. Viral infection.

Q297. A baker attends his occupational health department describing breathlessness and wheeze while at work. Which one of the following is the most appropriate next step?

a. Remove worker from workplace.
b. Blood testing.
c. Peak flow monitoring.
d. Spirometry.
e. Chest X-ray.

Q298. The production of the following foodstuffs is associated with occupational asthma except for which one?

a. Processed meat products.
b. Shrimp manufacture.
c. Mushrooms.
d. Bread.
e. Coffee.

Q299. A 35-year-old office worker is referred with worsening breathlessness. He is an ex-smoker, has a 10-pack/year history and continues to vape regularly. He has recently moved from the USA and his work colleagues complain about the sweet-smelling vaping fumes outside the office. His chest X-ray is normal, but he has markedly obstructive spirometry and is found to be hypoxic after walking from the carpark. He has never worked in a dusty environment and has never been exposed to any known respiratory sensitisers. Which one of the following is the most likely diagnosis?

a. Occupational asthma.
b. Hypersensitivity pneumonitis.

c. Silicosis.
d. Idiopathic pulmonary fibrosis (IPF).
e. Bronchiolitis obliterans ('popcorn lung').

Q300. Which one of the following occupational respiratory diseases is correctly paired with an at-risk occupation?

a. Emphysema (COPD) in cadmium workers.
b. Mesothelioma in electronics workers.
c. Asthma in pig farmers.
d. Silicosis in aircraft industry workers.
e. Tuberculosis in veterinarians.

Q301. Which one of the following is the best fit regarding recommending a vaccine in an otherwise well worker?

a. Flu vaccine in bus drivers.
b. Pneumococcal vaccine in welders.
c. Flu vaccine in poultry farmers.
d. Meningococcal vaccine in students.
e. Pneumococcal vaccine in healthcare workers.

Q302. Which one of the following is not a respiratory sensitiser?

a. Latex.
b. Enzymes.
c. Rat urine.
d. Ammonia.
e. Isocyanates.

Q303. A car mechanic has been referred with symptoms while painting cars in an enclosed workshop. His general practitioner has arranged peak flow monitoring and run the subsequent data through the Occupational Asthma expert SYStem (OASYS) database. Which one of the following OASYS scores is likely to be diagnostic of occupation-related symptoms?

a. OASYS score = 0.
b. OASYS score = 0.5.
c. OASYS score = 2.
d. OASYS score = 3.5.
e. None of the above.

Q304. As part of health surveillance on workers exposed to potentially high levels of respirable silica, which one of the following is correct?

a. All workers should be screened for tuberculosis.
b. All workers should have a high-resolution CT of chest.
c. Two sets of spirometry readings are an absolute minimum.
d. Only those with symptoms should having screening spirometry.
e. A fall in the predicted FVC below 80% should merit further investigation.

Q305. Which one of the following is the most common occupation to be diagnosed with occupational asthma in the UK?

a. Bakers.
b. Stainless steel welders.
c. Hairdressers.
d. Vehicle paint technicians.
e. Laboratory animal workers.

Q306. A cleaner with no prior respiratory history is referred with breathlessness and wheeze following a one-off significant exposure to fumes generated while incorrectly diluting a cleaning product in an enclosed storeroom. She has evidence of airflow obstruction on spirometry. Which one of the following is the best fit?

a. Occupational asthma secondary to sensitisation.
b. Irritant-induced asthma.
c. Reactive airways dysfunction syndrome (RADS).
d. Inducible laryngeal obstruction/vocal cord dysfunction.
e. None of the above.

Q307. A school laboratory technician is referred with cough and breathlessness. His symptoms started after he took over the role of looking after the cockroaches in the biology laboratories. The most likely diagnosis is which one of the following?

a. Hypersensitivity pneumonitis.
b. Irritant-induced asthma.
c. Pulmonary fibrosis.
d. Reactive airways dysfunction syndrome.
e. Occupational asthma.

Q308. Which one of the following does NOT increase the risk of developing lung cancer?

a. Asbestos exposure.
b. Prolonged radon exposure.
c. Exposure to respirable silica.
d. Working with asphalt.
e. Prolonged working with cadmium.

Q309. Several workers in a foundry are referred with fevers, cough and breathlessness. Their main job is cutting metal parts at a well-ventilated workstation with metal working fluid as a lubricant in the process. Which one of the following is the best fit diagnosis?

a. Hypersensitivity pneumonitis.
b. Occupational asthma secondary to sensitisation.
c. Irritant-induced asthma.
d. Reactive airways dysfunction syndrome.
e. None of the above.

Q310. A semi-professional ice hockey player is referred with breathlessness and wheeze while training on the ice rink. Which one of the following is the least likely diagnosis?

a. Carbon monoxide poisoning.
b. Hypersensitivity pneumonitis.

c. Exercise-induced bronchoconstriction.
d. Asthma.
e. Nitrogen dioxide poisoning.

Q311. All of the following cause hypersensitivity pneumonitis (HP) with the exception of which one?

a. Working with mushrooms.
b. Working with mouldy hay.
c. Working with popcorn sweeteners.
d. Working with pigeons.
e. Working with oysters.

Q312. All the following can produce occupational asthma in food workers with the exception of which one?

a. Sensitisation to wheat.
b. Sensitisation to enzymes.
c. Sensitisation to bleach cleaning products.
d. Sensitisation to coffee beans.
e. Sensitisation to spice mixes.

Q313. An electronics worker is referred with worsening breathlessness and cough. Her main role is soldering circuit boards. Peak flow monitoring is strongly suggestive of work-related asthma. Which one of the following is most likely to be responsible for this?

a. Colophony.
b. Beryllium.
c. Stainless steel.
d. Aluminium.
e. All of the above.

Q314. A 22-year-old bakery worker has confirmed sensitisation to alpha amylase with strongly positive peak flow monitoring in the workplace. In advising the employer, which one of the following is the best fit?

a. Strict occupational hygiene in the workplace to ensure workplace exposure limits are not exceeded.
b. Regular bronchodilator use prior to entering the workplace.
c. Redeployment.
d. Terminate the worker's employment due to ill health.
e. Maintenance of oral steroids.

Q315. A 55-year-old stone mason is referred with weight loss, breathlessness and persistent frank haemoptysis. He has a 60-pack/year smoking history and on examination, he has finger clubbing and is overtly cachectic. Which one of the following is the most likely diagnosis?

a. Chronic obstructive pulmonary disease (COPD).
b. Asbestosis.
c. Silicosis.
d. Idiopathic pulmonary fibrosis.
e. Primary lung cancer.

Q316. Which one of the non-smoking workers in the following occupations are at increased risk of developing chronic obstructive pulmonary disease (COPD)?

a. Sculptors.
b. Groundspeople/park keepers.
c. Food, drink and tobacco processors.
d. Plastic processors/moulders.
e. All of the above.

Q317. A health spa cleaner is referred with fevers breathlessness, wheeze and cough. He found his symptoms were worst when cleaning the jacuzzi tubs. Following a prolonged period of sick leave after his first day back at work, the fevers and respiratory symptoms recurred. Which one of the following is the most likely diagnosis?

a. Occupational asthma.
b. Occupational chronic obstructive pulmonary disease (COPD).
c. Acute hypersensitivity pneumonitis.
d. Irritant-induced asthma.
e. Idiopathic pulmonary fibrosis.

Q318. A shipyard worker is referred with breathless but normal spirometry. He is known to have pleural plaques on an old chest X-ray. He describes some right-sided pleuritic pain as well as marked weight loss. Clinically he has signs of a pleural effusion. The most likely diagnosis in this worker is which one of the following?

a. Chronic obstructive pulmonary disease (COPD).
b. Silicosis.
c. Pleural plaques.
d. Mesothelioma.
e. Asbestosis.

Q319. Which one of the following is the best fit in the causation of occupational asthma in hairdressers?

a. Para-phenylamine diamine-based dyes.
b. Henna.
c. Persulphate salt dyes.
d. Hairspray.
e. Perfumes.

Q320. Coal miners are at increased risk of the following conditions with the exception of which one of the following:

a. Coal worker's pneumoconiosis.
b. Chronic obstructive pulmonary disease (COPD).
c. Silicosis.
d. Tuberculosis.
e. Lung cancer.

Q321. The following conditions can be caused by repeated exposure to welding fume. Which one does NOT fit?

a. Metal fume fever.
b. Hypersensitivity pneumonitis.
c. Pulmonary fibrosis.
d. Bacterial pneumonia.
e. Chronic obstructive pulmonary disease (COPD).

Q322. An operative in a car seat manufacturing plant is referred with wheeze at work, strongly positive work peak flow testing and good response to asthma treatment initiated by the general practitioner. His employer is keen to see what may have caused his symptoms and whether he can continue to work in his job at the plant. Which one of the following tests is most likely to helpful?

a. Specific IgE to cat/dog dander.
b. Specific IgE to MDI/TDI isocyanates.
c. Specific IgE to dust mite.
d. CT scanning of chest.
e. None of the above, and he likely has irritant-induced asthma symptoms.

Q323. Which one of the following conditions is often associated with coal miners?

a. Systemic lupus erythematosus.
b. Rheumatoid arthritis.
c. Polymyalgia rheumatica.
d. Asthma.
e. Osteoarthritis.

Q324. The incidence of occupational asthma (OA) worldwide is in the region of 12–300 cases per million workers per annum, accounting for one in six cases of new-onset adult asthma. In that context, which one of the following statements is incorrect?

a. All adults with new-onset or reactivated childhood asthma should be asked their occupation and whether symptoms are better on days away from work and on holiday.
b. Persistent exposure to an asthmagen can lead to physiological decline, absenteeism and financial loss.
c. Favourable health and employment outcomes are achieved with rapid diagnosis and removal from exposure to or avoidance of causative agents.
d. Occupational asthma is routinely recognised by healthcare professionals.
e. Asthma is diagnosed by spirometry.

Skin Disorders

Q325. In regard to occupational dermatitis, which one of the following statements does NOT fit?

a. Occupations associated with it include engineering, hairdressing, woodworking and floristry.
b. In general, irritant contact dermatitis is more common than allergic contact dermatitis.
c. Previous history at pre-employment assessment is best indicator for future.
d. For the employee, personal economic issues can override preventive strategies.
e. Widespread use of barrier creams has led to a decrease in the incidence.

Q326. In the management of dermatitis, which one of the following statements does NOT fit?

a. The acute case should be removed from the source of exposure.
b. Alternative work is an option to explore.
c. A skin care policy may be of benefit.
d. Cationic skin cleansers are likely to cause skin reactions.
e. Solvents used as cleansers can be beneficial in removing oil and grease.

Q327. In regard to psoriasis, which one of the following statements does NOT fit?

a. It is characterised by dry, silvery scaling plaques and papules.
b. Sero-negative arthritis is a feature.
c. Occupational contact factors aggravate the condition.
d. Pruritus is common.
e. Catering work may be contraindicated.

Q328. In regard to photoallergic skin reactions, which one of the following is correct?

a. Have a different pathophysiology to allergic contact dermatitis.
b. Confirmation requires photo patch testing.
c. Are more common than phototoxic reactions.
d. Typically appear gradually on sun-exposed areas.
e. Do not appear on sun-exposed areas.

Q329. In regard to patch testing, which one of the following is the best fit?

a. Is typically used in the evaluation of irritant contact dermatitis.
b. Depends primarily on a type 1 immunological response to the agent.
c. Depends primarily on a type 4 delayed hypersensitivity response.
d. Is read after 24 hours.
e. Scarring may occur in 1 in 100,000 patch tests.

Q330. In relation to the Koebner phenomenon, whereby new skin lesions related to a pre-existing condition are triggered by traumatic injury to the skin, which one of the following statements is the best fit?

a. The phenomenon is well described in lichen planus.
b. It occurs less frequently during remission of psoriasis.
c. The phenomenon is well described in vitiligo.
d. It is a clinical feature of pityriasis rosea.
e. The phenomenon is well described in atopic eczema.

Q331. Allergic contact dermatitis (ACD) is a common occupational disease. Which one of the following statements is incorrect?

a. Hairdressers and beauticians are at increased risk of occupational chronic hand eczema.
b. ACD is a lymphocyte-mediated, delayed-type (type 4) hypersensitivity reaction which causes chronic pruritic dermatitis.
c. Definitive treatment of ACD is topical steroids.
d. ACD, particularly occupational ACD, has profound negative effects on quality of life and may lead to sickness absence, early retirement, loss of job or job change.
e. Early patch testing improves quality-of-life outcomes in hand eczema patients and has been shown to be cost effective.

Q332. In relation to skin cancer, which one of the following statements is the best fit?

a. Recent research has shown the attributable fraction for occupation in relation to cutaneous malignant melanoma in the UK is around 0.5%.

b. Sir Percivall Pott famously described soot warts in 1875 that led to scrotal cancer and triggered the Chimney Sweepers Act some years later.

c. Outdoor workers who have had organ transplants are at very high risk of squamous cell carcinoma (SCC).

d. Bowen's disease is the most common occupational skin carcinoma related to arsenic and is primarily work-related gastrointestinal exposure.

e. UVA penetrates deeper into the skin and is more important than UVB in carcinogenesis.

Match the following conditions to a causative agent:

Q333. Common cause of irritant contact dermatitis.

Q334. Oil folliculitis.

Q335. Occupational vitiligo.

Q336. Common cause of allergic contact dermatitis.

Q337. Chloracne.

a. Contact with polychlorinated aromatic hydrocarbons.
b. Hardwoods, epoxy resin, rubber, formaldehyde.
c. Result of irritation with mineral oil residues.
d. Detergents, solvents, cutting oils, cement.
e. Contact with alkyl phenols.

Match the following with the correct response:

Q338. A skin irritant.

Q339. Patch testing.

Q340. A skin allergen.

Q341. Photocontact dermatitis.

Q342. Contact urticaria.

a. Wheal and flare response sometimes found in hairdressers and animal handlers.
b. Provocation of contact dermatitis with stimulus of ultraviolet rays.
c. Use of test agents in allergic contact dermatitis.
d. An agent that directly damages cells if applied in sufficient concentration or for sufficient time.
e. An agent that induces a specific immunological sensitivity to itself.

Q343. In regard to workplace skin disease occurring in clusters, which one of the following is incorrect?

a. Allergic contact dermatitis.
b. Pityriasis rosea.
c. A functional phenomenon.
d. Photodermatitis.
e. Vitiligo.

Toxicology, Metals and Solvents

Q344. The effects of long-term exposure to volatile anaesthetics on healthcare personnel can cause harm. Regarding waste anaesthetic gases, which one of the following statements is the best fit?

a. There is no evidence of adverse effects when environmental levels are kept within legal threshold values.
b. There is good evidence for an increase in spontaneous abortions when scavenging devices are not used.
c. There is good evidence for an increase in congenital abnormalities when scavenging devices are not used.
d. Halothane is a potent hepatotoxin which is still widely used.
e. Post-anaesthetic recovery rooms pose minimal exposure risk.

Q345. In relation to the properties of arsenic, which one of the following statements is the best fit?

a. Organic arsenic is more toxic than inorganic arsenic.
b. Pentavalent arsenic is more toxic than its trivalent form.
c. It is readily absorbed through intact skin.
d. It is moderately absorbed from the gut.
e. Crustaceans and other fish are a known source of organic arsenic exposure; however, in this form, the toxicity is considered to be negligible.

Q346. In regard to the effects of chemicals on the body, which one of the following statements is incorrect?

a. Corrosive: a chemical that causes visible destruction of, or irreversible alterations in, living tissue by chemical action at the site of contact.
b. Irritant: a chemical that is not corrosive but that causes reversible inflammatory effects on living tissue at the site of contact.
c. Mutagen: a chemical that causes birth defects.
d. Sensitiser: a chemical that will cause an allergic reaction in a substantial number of exposed people.
e. Carcinogen: a chemical that causes or potentially causes cancer.

Q347. In regard to significant hydrofluoric acid (HF) exposure, which one of the following is the best fit?

a. Hypercalcemia.
b. Hypokalemia.
c. Metabolic alkalosis.
d. Prolonged QT on ECG.
e. Immediate treatment with calcium phosphate.

Q348. In regard to LD50, which one of the following statements does NOT fit?

a. The LD50 is a measure of acute toxicity.
b. The LD50 is the dose of a test chemical that causes death in 50% of exposed lab animals.
c. The LD50 is the lethal concentration of an aerosol, gas, vapour or particulate that, when administered to a group of test animals by inhalation, causes death in 50% of those animals.
d. The LD50 results vary depending on the route of exposure.
e. The LD50 results vary depending on the test animal species used.

Q349. In regard to aliphatic organic compounds, which one of the following does NOT fit?

a. Carbon disulphide.
b. Carbon tetrachloride.
c. Chloroform.
d. Benzene.
e. Formaldehyde.

Q350. In regard to hepatotoxicity, which one of the following does NOT fit?

a. Tetrachloroethane.
b. Tetrachloroethylene.
c. Monochloroethylene.
d. Carbon tetrachloride.
e. Polyvinyl chloride.

Q351. In dose-response relationships, the term 'threshold' refers to which one of the following?

a. The dose at which no observable adverse effect occurs.
b. The interval of time between exposure and development of the health effect.
c. The dose below which the probability of an individual responding is 0.
d. The dose of substance that can be expected to cause death in 50% of exposed.
e. The degree to which a substance exhibits a dose-response relationship.

Q352. Nanotoxicology, a relatively new field of science and technology, is the branch of toxicology which deals with risks imposed by engineered nanoparticles (NPs). Which one of the following statements is the best fit?

a. NPs can be found naturally in the environment.
b. Artificial nanomaterials can be synthesised by grinding.
c. Particles with any dimension measuring less than 100 nm are classified as nanoparticles.
d. Particle behaviour differs from that of bulk material due to smaller particle size, surface effects and quantum effects.
e. Nanostructured objects are likely to be hazardous to human health.

Match the following agents with their properties:

Q353. Vapours.

Q354. Fumes.

Q355. Mists.

Q356. Aerosols.

a. Solid particles generated by condensation from the gaseous state, generally after volatilisation from molten metals.
b. Liquid droplets or solid particles dispersed in air of a fine enough particle size to remain dispersed for some time.
c. Gaseous form of a substance normally solid or liquid which occurs by the process of evaporation.
d. Suspended droplets generated by condensation from gaseous to liquid state or the breaking up of a liquid into a dispersed state.

Match the following substances with their monitoring agents:

Q357. Lead.

Q358. Trichloroethylene.

Q359. Vinyl chloride monomer.

Q360. Benzene.

Q361. Xylene.

a. Urinary thiodiglycolic acid.
b. Urinary methyl hippuric acid.
c. Urinary trichloroacetic acid.
d. Urinary ALA.
e. Urinary phenols.

Match the following poisons with their sign/symptoms:

Q362. Lead poisoning.

Q363. Mercury poisoning.

Q364. Cadmium poisoning.

Q365. Chromium poisoning.

Q366. Manganese poisoning.

a. Brown-blue line on gums, fulminant itch, erethism, cerebellar cortical atrophy and dislocation of lens.
b. Skin ulceration, pneumonitis, asthma and lung cancer.
c. Respiratory irritation, organic psychosis and Parkinsonism.
d. Abdominal pain, anaemia, raised erythrocyte protoporphyrin and siderocytes in peripheral blood.
e. Focal emphysema, anosmia, renal calculi and glycosuria.

Q367. Green discoloration of the tongue is a characteristic of exposure to which one of the following?

a. Mercury.
b. Vanadium.

c. Zinc.
d. Lead.
e. Iodine.

Q368. In relation to vanadium, which one of the following is correct?

a. Elemental vanadium is present crude oil.
b. Vanadium is a probable human carcinogen.
c. Vanadium pentoxide is a potent hepatic toxin.
d. Vanadium pentoxide is a skin sensitiser.
e. Exposure can be associated with respiratory tract toxicity.

Q369. When considering aluminium, which one of the following statements is the best fit?

a. The Hall–Héroult process for refining aluminium can release chlorine from the electrolytic process that causes worker respiratory function problems.
b. Workers involved in recycling metals, including aluminium, can be exposed to dioxins when grease and coatings are burnt off.
c. Mild cognitive decline is 5.5 times more likely in aluminium smelters after more than 10 years of exposure, compared with the general population.
d. Whereas bauxite is considered to be reasonably inert contamination, beryllium remains a significant risk for respiratory complications.
e. Increased telangiectasia in aluminium smelters is associated with increased cardiovascular disease independent of smoking.

Q370. In regard to cadmium, which one of the following is the best fit?

a. Cadmium has a higher melting point than most of the metals it is alloyed with, therefore low concentrations are produced when oxyacetylene cutting or smelting takes place and long periods of exposure are required to have an effect.
b. Cigarette smoke is an important source of environmental cadmium and smokers have higher liver concentrations of cadmium, which affects urine screening thresholds.
c. Carcinogenicity is recognised by IARC who classify cadmium as a Group 2 agent.
d. Cadmium accumulates in the kidneys and the liver and this triggers renal production of the cadmium-metallothionein complex which excretes via the kidneys.
e. Does not have any respiratory tract toxicity.

Q371. In regard to elemental mercury, which one of the following is the best fit?

a. Is an essential element in humans.
b. Has a low vapour pressure.
c. Is efficiently absorbed after ingestion.
d. Readily crosses the placenta.
e. Is well absorbed in the gastrointestinal tract.

Q372. In regard to chromium (Cr), which one of the following is the best fit?

a. Toxicity is usually due to the Cr III compounds.
b. Biological monitoring typically by pre-shift measurement of chromium in urine.
c. Is a soft silver metal.
d. Toxicity usually due to the Cr VI compounds.
e. Inhalation results in an increased risk of lung cancer.

Q373. A 45-year-old metal plate worker presents with a persistent nasal discharge. His nasal septum has a reddened ulcerated area. Which one of the following exposures best supports the diagnosis of chrome-induced ulcer?

a. Trivalent chromium.
b. Chromic oxide.
c. Chromic sulphate.
d. Hexavalent chromium salts.
e. Chromium telluride.

Q374. The chemical formula for toluene is which one of the following?

a. $C2H5OH$.
b. $C7H8$.
c. $C8H9$.
d. $C8O9$.
e. $C7OH$.

Q375. When considering the properties of toluene, which one of the following is the best fit?

a. Is an aromatic hydrocarbon.
b. Is an aliphatic hydrocarbon.
c. Is a hydrocarbon.
d. Mixes well with water.
e. Is denser than water.

Q376. When considering the properties of xylene, which one of the following is the best fit?

a. Is a known human carcinogen.
b. Is poorly absorbed through skin.
c. Is a major constituent of petrol/gasoline.
d. Has broadly similar toxicological effects as toluene.
e. Is banned in Europe due to its toxicity.

Q377. Which one of the following is not a 'stochastic event'?

a. Sensitisation.
b. Carcinogenesis.
c Teratogenicity.
d. Mutagenesis.
e. Chromosomal aberrations.

chapter 02

DOI: 10.1201/9781003291930-02

Modified Essay Questions (MEQs)

MEQ1. You are providing clinical supervision and support for a mass vaccination clinic and are called to assess someone who feels unwell post vaccination:

Q378. What are the possible diagnoses?

Q379. You assess the patient who is conscious but feels unwell. What signs and symptoms may help you to clarify whether this is anaphylaxis?

Q380. You suspect anaphylaxis. What is your management of this?

Q381. The patient remains unwell five minutes later. What is your management protocol in this situation?

Q382. Eventually the patient begins to feel better. Outline your management of the patient and the situation.

MEQ2. You work as an occupational health consultant, and you are asked to advise a local car body repair business about the risks to health associated with car body spray painting.

Q383. What potentially toxic agent may be of significance in this process?

Q384. What type of health effect would you be most concerned about?

Q385. What types of control measures would you look for?

Q386. Outline the type of health surveillance that should be carried out in this context.

Q387. What tests may be useful in diagnosing occupational asthma?

Q388. Give three examples of high-risk occupations and associated agent.

Q389. What advice would you give someone diagnosed with occupational asthma?

MEQ3. You are a specialist occupational physician working with a company providing consultancy services to large corporate enterprises. The HR Manager of an insurance company is concerned about a growing number of complaints from employees regarding symptoms they associate with their working environment, specifically their perception of poor air quality in the building. Most of the 300 employees work in open plan, air-conditioned offices in a building they have occupied for 20 years. They report that they are suffering from sick building syndrome (SBS).

Q390. What are the two main health complaints reported by employees in this situation?

Q391. Name three physical factors known to contribute to the phenomenon.

Q392. What initial questions might you ask before arranging a more detailed exploration of the problem?

Q393. What are the potential chemical air contaminants in an office environment?

MEQ4. You are a specialist occupational physician providing services to a large care home. Pauline is a 35-year-old nurse assistant who has been referred for assessment as she has been off sick for two weeks with back pain. The pain came on some hours after a 10-hour shift, and she recalls a 'twinge' whilst manoeuvring a particularly heavy patient into a hoist. She complains bitterly of pain in the right lumbar region radiating on occasion to the buttock. She has a constant aching pain which is aggravated by 'any movement' as well as prolonged sitting or standing. She is 'crippled' in the morning upon rising and her whole leg has 'given way' on three occasions. The pain at its worst is 'more than 10' on a visual analogue scale (VAS). Her general practitioner has advised her to 'take it easy', and he is making plans for an MRI in the local private hospital. She generally does not take tablets but is taking paracetamol periodically. She lives with her aged mother who has recently been diagnosed with dementia. She smokes 20 cigarettes a day and has become somewhat house-bound (apart from work) because of her mother's needs. She enjoys work but had a 'row' with her superior on the morning of her last day at work. She expresses anxiety about losing her job if her back does not recover. You notice she has an antalgic gait and is holding her right loin region while walking. She is anxious and fearful of examination. Her lumbar range of movement is severely limited in all planes. She grimaces and moans whilst getting on the examination couch. She has a positive straight leg raise on the RHS at 30 degrees and leg raise is limited on the left at 45 degrees but with no pain. SLR of 90 degrees is achieved while seated upright. Axial loading test is positive. Sacroiliac distraction test is positive on the RHS. There is no demonstrable myotomal weakness, impairment of reflexes or sensory loss. There is generalised tenderness over the right lumbar area, but this is more marked overlying the sacroiliac joint.

Q394. What is the likely nature of her back pain?

Q395. Identify three further questions you would like to ask related to current symptoms to exclude red flags.

Q396. Identify three further questions you would like to ask as part of the medical history to exclude red flags.

Q397. What yellow flags are worth exploring in this case?

Q398. Is there evidence of behavioural symptoms and overt pain behaviour? If so, please identify and comment on significance.

Q399. Does she demonstrate behavioural signs? If so, what is their significance?

Q400. Does she require any investigation at this stage?

Q401. Does she require medication or other advice on managing her symptoms?

MEQ5. A theatre nurse presents to the occupational health department after sustaining a needlestick injury from a known patient during theatre, the previous day.

Q402. What infectious diseases are usually considered for blood and bodily fluid exposures in healthcare?

Q403. How would you manage the case?

Q404. What infectious diseases have an efficacious post-exposure prophylactic treatment and what are the timelines for initiating same?

MEQ6. During a pre-placement health assessment, a healthcare worker recently arrived in Ireland from India has a positive interferon gamma release assay result.

Q405. What are the differential diagnoses?

Q406. How would you proceed?

Q407. What are the implications on fitness for duty?

MEQ7. You provide occupational health advice to a metal fabrication workshop. A 55-year-old worker presents complaining of ringing in both ears and gradually disimproving hearing.

Q408. How would you initially manage this issue?

Q409. What investigations may be useful?

Q410. His audiogram reveals a bilateral hearing loss sloping down in the higher frequencies with a notch at 4 kHz. What is the most likely diagnosis and what other diagnoses would you consider?

Q411. What types of control measures would you look for in a workplace assessment?

Q412. What other measures are important?

Q413. What advice would you give?

MEQ8. You work as an occupational health specialist with the health service. A nurse presents to you with bilateral hand dermatitis, predominantly affecting the web spaces between the fingers.

Q414. What is the most likely diagnosis and what other diagnoses would you consider?

Q415. What are the possible causes of this health problem in nurses?

Q416. How would you initially manage this issue? Are there other health effects that may cause concern?

Q417. What types of control measures would you look for?

Q418. You review the nurse three weeks later and the problem has not improved. How would you now proceed with managing the case?

Q419. What advice would you give someone diagnosed with occupational dermatitis?

MEQ9. A 40-year-old general operative in a factory presents to the occupational health centre complaining of low back pain. He stated that it developed one hour prior to presenting after

lifting a 20 kg box from the floor. He stated that the pain was mainly across his lower back and that it did not radiate to the legs.

Q420. Low back pain can be categorised into three categories. Can you name them?

Q421. What is the likely diagnosis in this case?

Q422. What treatment would you consider?

Q423. What would you advise in regard to fitness for duty?

Q424. What would you advise the Environmental, Health and Safety Department?

MEQ10. An employee has been referred to occupational health as she was certified unfit for duty by her general practitioner with a diagnosis of work-related stress.

Q425. How would you define work-related stress?

Q426. What are the UK Health and Safety Executive Management Standards?

Q427. What potential treatment and supports are appropriate in such a case?

Q428. What are the potential outcomes that could form the confidential medical report back to the referring manager?

MEQ11. An employee working from home contacts his occupational health service complaining of sore eyes. The role involves computer work, with multiple meetings online daily. Before the COVID-19 pandemic, the employee worked in the office with colleagues and attended meetings face to face.

Q429. What is the likely diagnosis?

Q430. What are the suggested treatments?

MEQ12. A 60-year-old woman presents in your clinic with a history of rash involving her hands, forearms and upper part of her chest. She works in a hatchery and cleans chick trays for most of her shift. She denies a previous history of skin problems.

Q431. What information further do you want from her?

Q432. She produces a piece of paper with the list of four substances she uses in her cleaning. You recognise two sensitisers and two irritants on the list. What are the options for diagnosis?
You see the woman the following year. She tells you she was moved away from the cleaning work to chick grading. She had a patch test last year and everything was negative except nickel. She is worried because her rash had cleared up not long after being moved. But now she has a rash on her forearm for the last month. The room is too warm for her because she gets hot flushes, so she has moved to wearing short-sleeved shirts. The grading area has all stainless-steel surfaces. She leans on the surface for long periods as she works.

Q433. What considerations might there be about her work surface and her nickel allergy?

MEQ13. You meet a doctor for a pre-placement medical who has moved to your hospital from a different region of the UK. They inform you they are HIV positive.

Q434. What details do you wish to establish as part of your initial assessment?

Q435. You establish they are a specialist registrar in AED, they are registered with UKAP-OHR and have a copy of their last report to UKAP-OHR, their last blood tests were five months ago and they have never been involved in EPPs. What do you do next?

Q436. The doctor is re-registered with UKAP-OHR and their first two viral load results are undetectable. Their next viral load returns as 300 cp/m. The doctor states they are well and compliant with anti-viral regimen. They had a mild COVID-19 infection three weeks ago. How do you manage this situation?

MEQ14. You assess a woman for a driving medical. She tells you she delivers goods to retail outlets and drives a 10 T lorry. Two weeks prior, she had coughing episode while at home and passed out, falling to the floor. The episode was witnessed and had no seizure features.

Q437. What advice do you give her about driving?

Q438. Her doctor tells her the cough was due to acid reflux and treats her successfully with a PPI. Eight weeks later and her reflux and cough have settled. She wants to return to driving. What advice do you give her?

Q439. The woman reveals that she has diabetes that is treated with insulin, and she has noticed that the warning symptoms of hypoglycaemia have diminished. Her doctor advised her to use a flash glucose monitoring system, and this has worked very well in alerting her if her glucose drops. She has not had an episode of severe hypoglycaemia. What does she need from a diabetes perspective to keep driving on a Group P2/vocational licence?

MEQ15. You receive a phone call to your NHS Occupational Health clinic informing you of several cases of pertussis in the Paediatric AED. You are asked to deal with potential workforce contacts.

Q440. What group is most at risk?

Q441. Which employees are you interested in for post-exposure assessment?

Q442. When is chemoprophylaxis advisable for healthcare workers?

Q443. When is vaccination advisable for pertussis after an incident?

chapter 03

DOI: 10.1201/9781003291930-03

Observed Structured Practical Examination Questions (OSPEs)

OSPE Station 1. A 35-year-old woman has been referred to your clinic for pre-employment health assessment pending her appointment as a cleaner at your hospital. She presents the results of bloods (Figure 3.1) taken prior to her departure from her home country (Eastern Europe) from where she has recently travelled. She is in good health.

SPECIMEN TYPE: SERUM TESTS	RESULT
Assay for HBsAg (Architect)	POSITIVE
Hepatitis B eAg (Architect)	NEGATIVE
Hepatitis B eAb (Architect)	POSITIVE
Hepatitis B core IgM antibody	NEGATIVE
EIA for Delta IgM (Diasorin)	NEGATIVE

FIGURE 3.1 OSPE Station 1.

Q444. How would you interpret the viral markers in Figure 3.1 and comment on their significance?

Q445. What other blood tests might be useful in clarifying her diagnosis further?

Q446. Is she fit for work?

Q447. If a prospective employee of the same age, gender and serology and with, in addition, an HBV DNA viral load of 2.3×10^4 IU/ml, attended for assessment, would you consider her fit to work as a general surgeon?

Q448. Explain the rationale for your decision.

Q449. Should this doctor be given treatment for her infection?

OSPE Station 2. A healthcare worker (HCW) calls the occupational health department 24 hours after receiving his first dose of a COVID-19 vaccination. He informs you that he has just developed a temperature of 39°C with fatigue at work. He advises you that he had a previous COVID-19 Detected PCR result 11 weeks prior. You refer him urgently for a COVID-19 PCR swab and advise him to self-isolate until the result is known. The result is processed in the local laboratory and the result states COVID-19 RNA detected.

Q450. What are the differential diagnoses?

Q451. How would you differentiate between a re-infection and a false positive result?

OSPE Station 3. A general operative in a medical device manufacturing factory presented to the occupational health physician complaining of right wrist pain of gradual onset over the preceding three to four months. His role involves polishing titanium orthopaedic implants using a rotating nylon wheel. Essentially, he is exposed to hand–arm vibration. He is in the role for 12 months. He does not rotate tasks.

Q452. What other symptoms would you ask for during the consultation?

Q453. What workplace factors would you enquire about?

Q454. What non-work-related factors would you enquire about?

The employee informs you that the only symptom is right wrist pain. He stated that it is aggravated by his work task. There is no occupational hygiene report available in regard to hand–arm vibration exposure. There is no evidence of a systemic rheumatological disorder. Physical examination is unremarkable.

Q455. What would your opinion be regarding fitness for work?

Q456. What initial treatment would you consider?

Q457. What other relevant input would you advise?

Q458. How would you manage the case going forward?

Q459. What would your approach to return to work be?

OSPE Station 4. A student nurse presents with inflamed palms and a history of two months after commencing placement on a hospital ward developed a rash on both hands and states that she thinks it is caused by alcohol gel hand sanitiser. Due to COVID-19 hygiene precautions she uses this repeatedly during the working day. She says it stings her hands when she applies some.

Q460. What is the differential diagnosis?

Q461. What are the salient points you would want to elicit from the worker?

Q462. What type of allergic reaction causes contact allergic dermatitis?

Q463. What type of allergic reaction causes urticaria?

Q464. Which occurs more commonly, contact irritant dermatitis or contact allergic dermatitis?

Q465. What is the likely cause of this rash if the diagnosis is contact irritation?

Q466. How would you manage a case of contact irritant dermatitis such as this?

Q467. Are there any infection prevention and control concerns in such a case?

Q468. What test is used to identify the allergen in contact allergic dermatitis?

OSPE Station 5. At the clinical OSPE station, a patient presents with a painful stiff shoulder.

Q469. Briefly outline the steps you would take in the clinical assessment of a shoulder joint.

OSPE Station 6. The results shown in Figure 3.2 are presented to you at an OSPE station. They belong to a 55-year-old heating engineer who is a smoker. You are asked to assess the findings and respond to the following questions:

Spirometry	Pre (L)	Pred (L)	% Pred	Z Score
FEV1	1.33	2.13	63	-2.73
FVC	1.54	2.49	62	-3.00
FEV1/FVC	86.38	86.38	102	0.33
PEFR	234.71	298.74	79	-1.05

Lung Vols	Pre (L)	Pred (L)	% Pred	Z Score
RV-He L	0.56	0.88	63	-1.55
FRC – He L	1.21	1.61	75	-1.40
TLC -He L	2.1	3.44	62	-3.82

Gas Transfer	Pre	Predicted	%Predicted
DLCO (SB) mmol/min/kPa	3.04	6.52	47
KCO mmol/min/kPa	1.47		
Hb (g/100ml)		12	

FIGURE 3.2 OSPE Station 6.

Q470. What clinical findings might be present?

Q471. How would you approach the assessment of the case?

Q472. What exposures may be associated with this type of picture?

OSPE Station 7. The X-ray image shown in Figure 3.3 is presented to you at an OSPE station. They belong to a 45-year-old builder who is a non-smoker. You are asked to assess the findings and respond to the following questions:

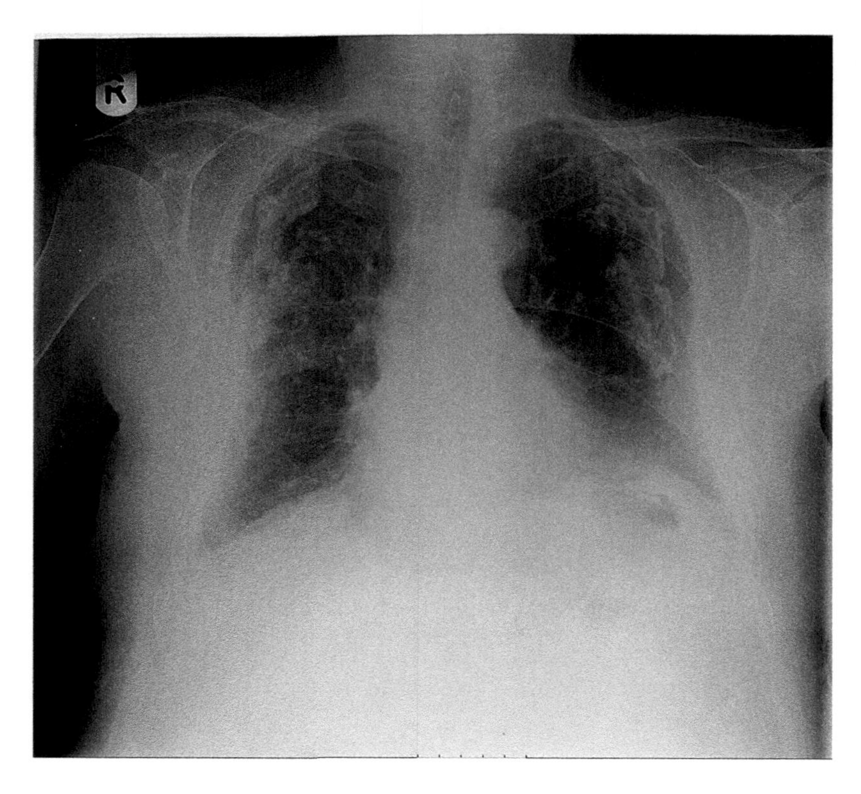

FIGURE 3.3 OSPE Station 7.

Q473. What is represented in the radiological images in Figure 3.3?

Q474. How would you approach the assessment of the case?

Q475. What advice would you give the patient?

OSPE Station 8. The instrument shown in Figure 3.4 is presented at the OSPE station.

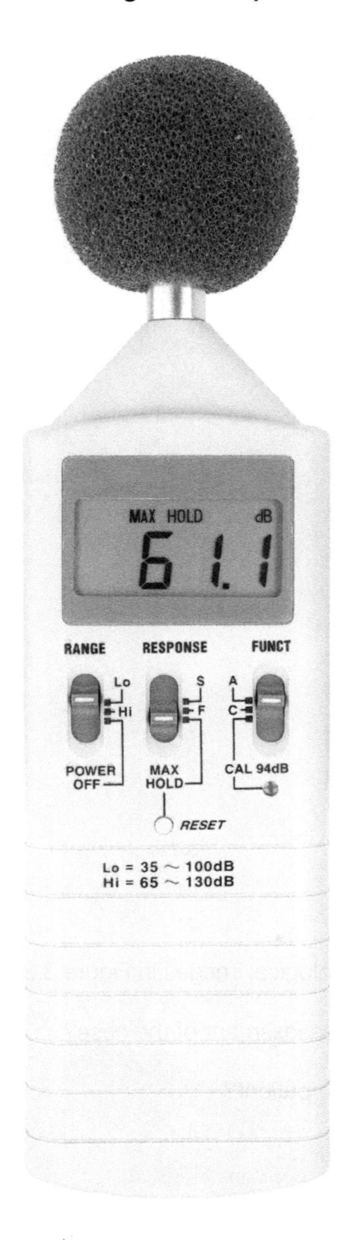

FIGURE 3.4 OSPE Station 8.

Q476. What is this instrument?

Q477. What is it used for in an OH setting?

Q478. Why is there a circular globe on the top?

OSPE Station 9. You are presented with the photograph shown in Figure 3.5 at the OSPE station. Answer the following questions:

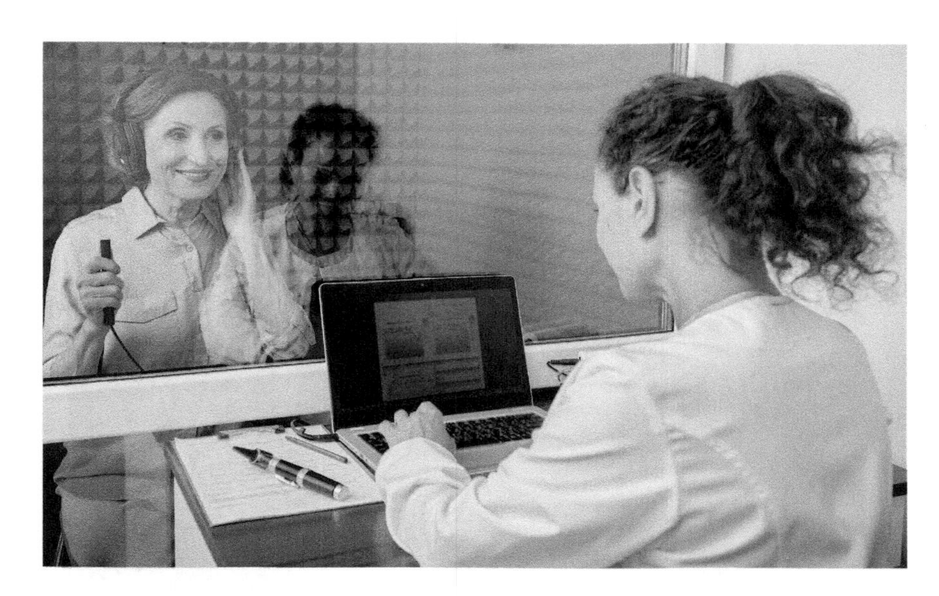

FIGURE 3.5 OSPE Station 9.

Q479. What is shown in the photograph?

Q480. When might this be performed?

OSPE Station 10. You are presented with the piece of equipment shown in Figure 3.6 at the OSPE station. Answer the following questions:

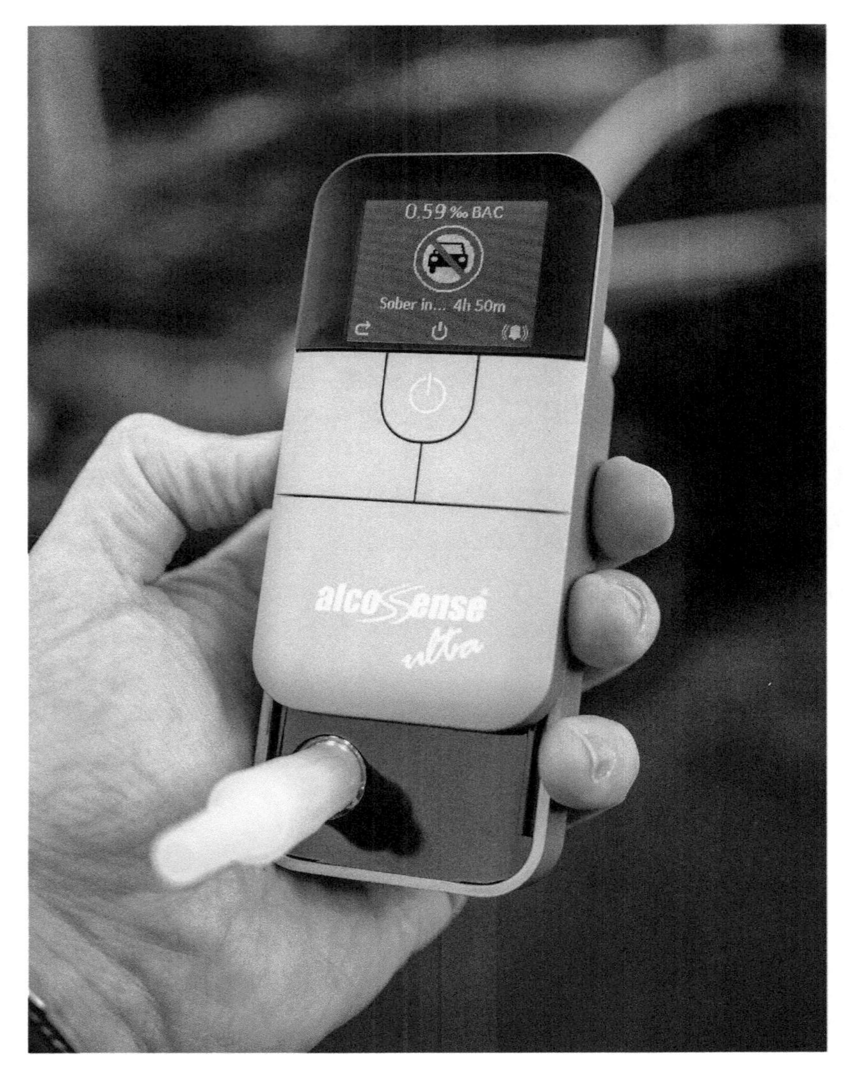

FIGURE 3.6 OSPE Station 10.

Q481. What is this piece of equipment?

Q482. What is it used for?

Q483. When might it be used in an OH setting?

OSPE Station 11. You are presented with the piece of equipment shown in Figure 3.7 at the OSPE station. Answer the following questions:

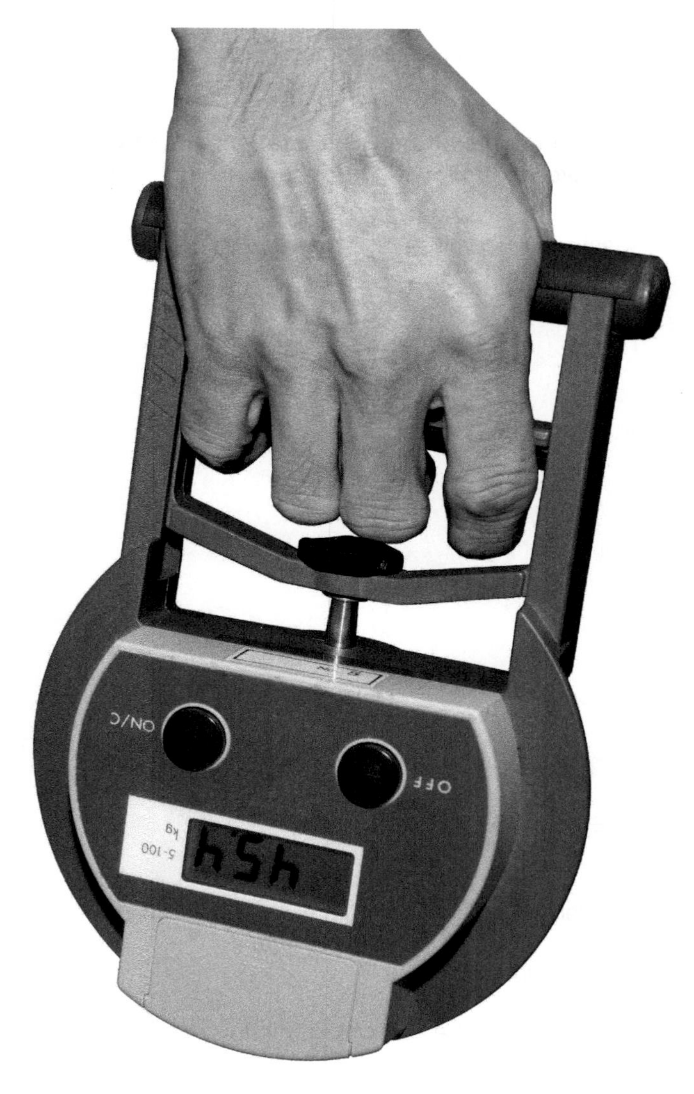

FIGURE 3.7 OSPE Station 11.

Q484. What is this piece of equipment?

Q485. What does it measure?

Q486. How is it used in an OH setting?

Q487. What are the main practical uses?

OSPE Station 12. A patient is presented at this clinical OSPE station who works as a factory operative in a meat-packing plant. He has been complaining of right knee pain on walking for the last four months. There is no other past medical history.

Q488. Briefly describe how you would examine the knee joint of this patient.

OSPE Station 13. The patient presents at the OSPE station with fingernails as shown in the photograph (Figure 3.8). Answer the following questions:

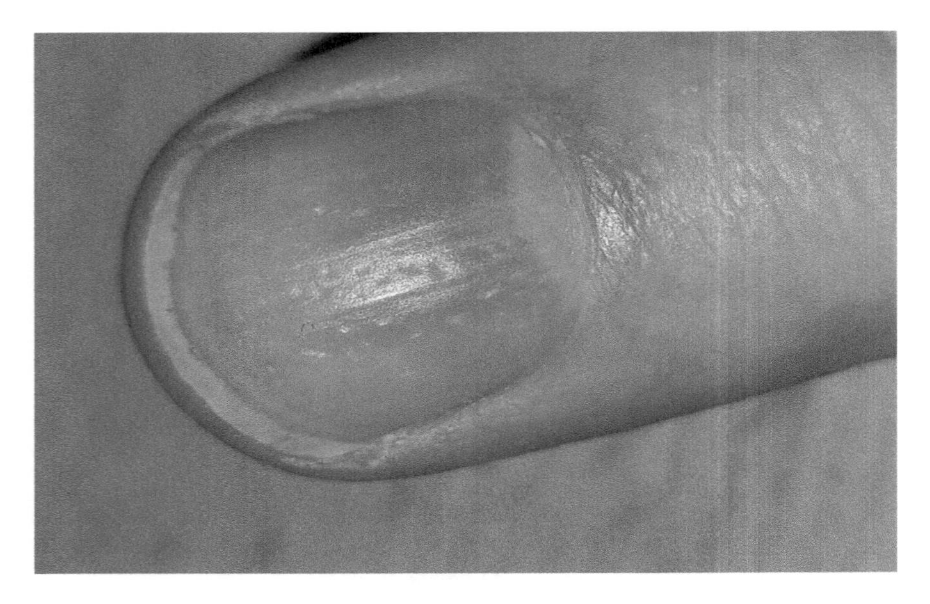

FIGURE 3.8 OSPE Station 13.

Q489. What nail lesion is evident in the photograph?

Q490. What is the most likely diagnosis?

Q491. Name other nail lesions that may be associated with this condition.

OSPE Station 14. The following X-ray image (Figure 3.9) of a male patient is presented at the OSPE station. The information given includes that the man presented at work with a history of stumbling, leg weakness and stiffness. He had no pain. He worked with a lot of solvents and occasionally acrylamide. Answer the following questions:

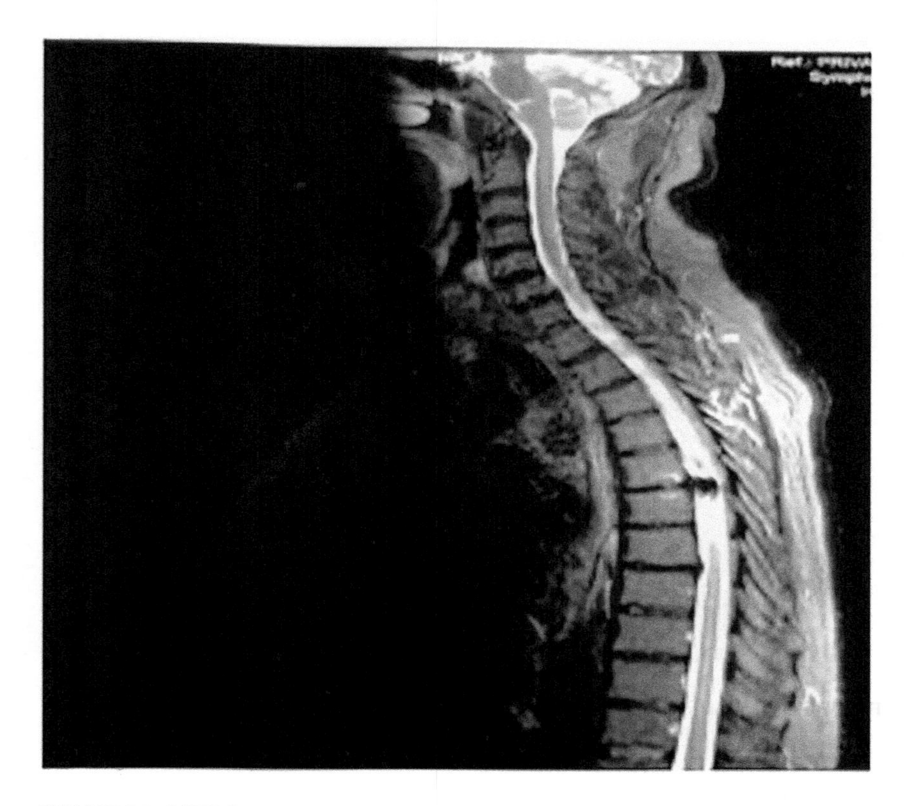

FIGURE 3.9 OSPE Station 14.

Q492. What type of X-ray is it?

Q493. Describe what you see in the X-ray.

OSPE Station 15. A patient is presented at this clinical OSPE station who works as a secretary in an office. She has been complaining of lower back pain for six months. There is no other past medical history.

Q494. Briefly describe how you would examine the lumbar spine of this patient.

OSPE Station 16. You are presented with the piece of equipment shown in Figure 3.10 at the OSPE station. Answer the following questions:

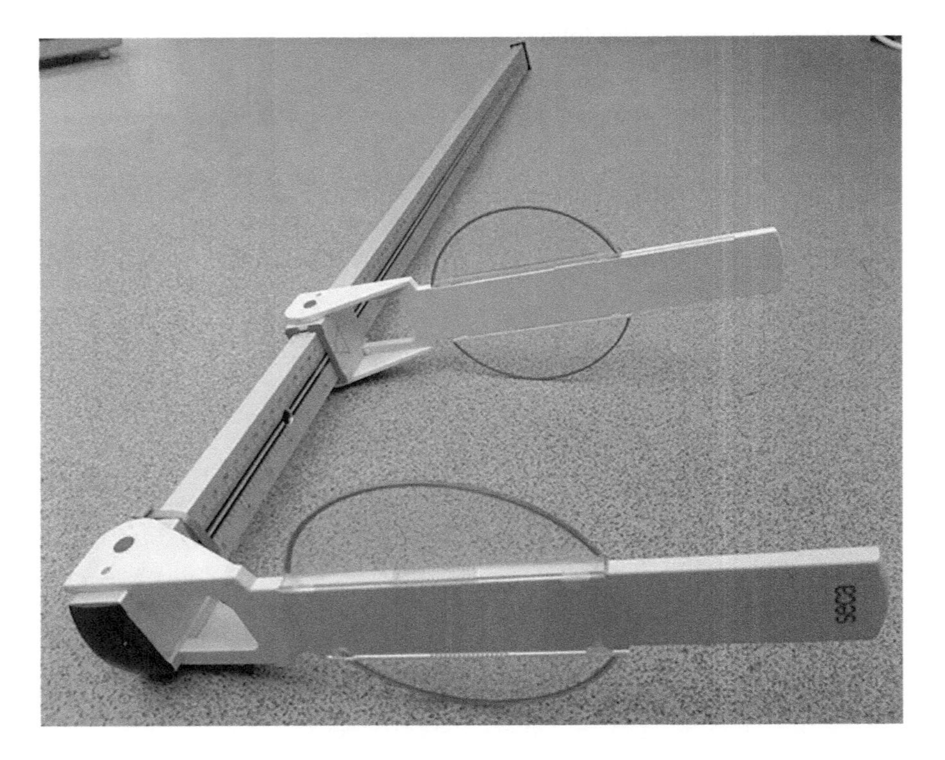

FIGURE 3.10 OSPE Station 16.

Q495. What is this equipment used for?

Q496. Why may it save lives?

OSPE Station 17. You are presented with the photograph shown in Figure 3.11 at the OSPE station. Answer the following questions:

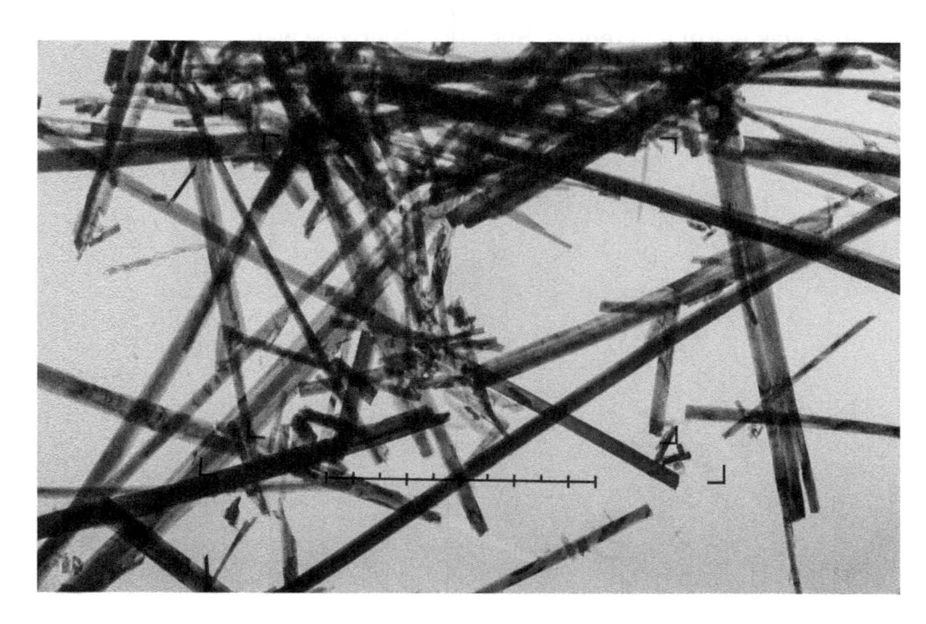

FIGURE 3.11 OSPE Station 17.

Q497. What is shown in the photograph?

Q498. What health effects are associated with exposure to the items in the picture?

Q499. What advice would you give someone exposed to these?

OSPE Station 18. A patient is presented at this clinical OSPE station who is a laboratory worker who handles small animals. He is a smoker and has been complaining of a wheezy chest for over 12 months. There is no other past medical history.

Q500. Briefly describe how you would examine the respiratory system of this patient.

OSPE Station 19. A photograph (Figure 3.12) of a patient's left shoulder is presented. You are given the history that the presentation is that of a skin reaction which occurred six days after the healthcare worker received her first dose of an mRNA COVID-19 vaccination. The erythematous area was warm and tender. She was otherwise well.

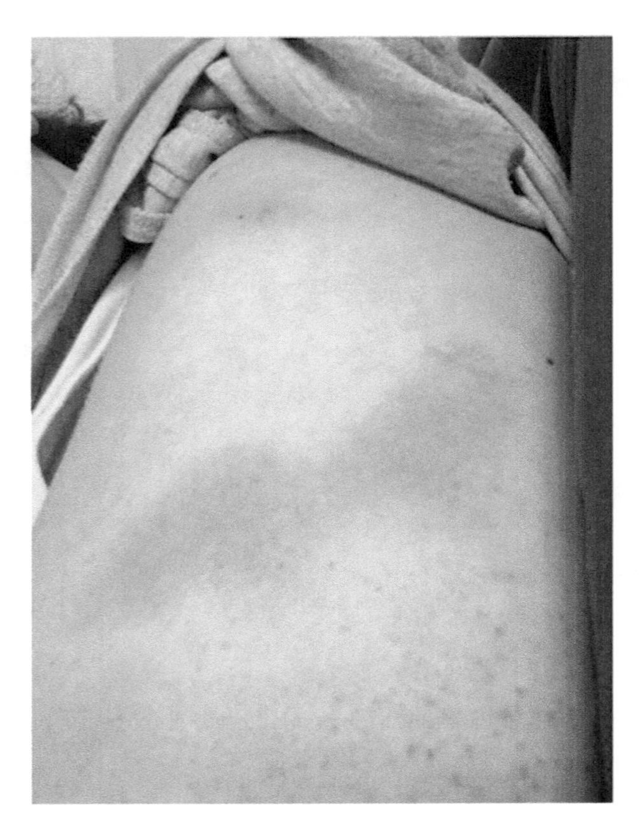

FIGURE 3.12 OSPE Station 19.

Q501. How would you approach the examination of the shoulder?

Q502. What is the likely diagnosis/explanation?

Q503. What would you advise as treatment?

Q504. Is the second dose of vaccination contraindicated in this case?

Image Acknowledgements

Figures 1, 2, 3, 8, 9, 10, 12: publication contributors.
Figure 4: BaLL LunLa/Shutterstock.com.
Figure 5: Peakstock/Shutterstock.com.
Figure 6: AlcoSense Laboratories, Maidenhead, UK.
Figure 7: WatcharesHansawek/Shutterstock.com.
Figure 11: Pvince/Shutterstock.com.

chapter 04

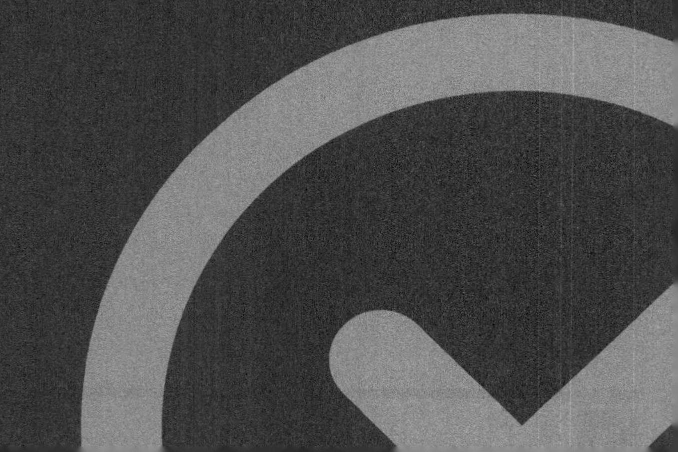

DOI: 10.1201/9781003291930-04

Answers

Multiple Choice Questions (MCQs)

Aviation and Diving

A1. (c). Divers who have dived low enough to exceed 1 bar are advised to delay flights because of the risk of DCS on commercial flights.

A2. (c). Best fit. The exosphere is the atmospheric layer furthest from the Earth. Hypoxia arising at increasing altitude is a direct consequence of a decrease in atmospheric pressure with consequent reduction of oxygen tension but not in the relative concentration of oxygen to other gases. With every 1,000 feet ascent, the temperature drops by 1.98°C. Commercial airlines confine themselves to the troposphere while certain military aircraft may operate within the stratospheric layer.

A3. (a). Best fit. Insidious effects of acute hypoxia may occur below 10,000 feet and include impairment of night vision, narrowing of peripheral vision and mild psychomotor and memory impairment. Cabin pressurisation achieves adequate levels of oxygen for passengers and crew. Military aircraft cannot be pressurised to the same degree as commercial aircraft without compromising manoeuvrability. Significant physical, cognitive and psychological impairment, including loss of judgement and decision-making capabilities, euphoria, sensory loss and incoordination occur at higher altitudes (greater than 10,000 feet).

A4. (a). Best fit. Ear, nose and throat (ENT) are the most frequent causes of grounding, with musculoskeletal and psychiatric the next most frequent. However, many ENT causes are temporary, whereas rarer cardiovascular and neurological may lead to prolonged and permanent grounding.

A5. (c). Recompression therapy is the administration of 100% oxygen in a sealed chamber for several hours. The chamber is pressurised to greater than 1 atmosphere and then gradually lowered to atmospheric pressure. In divers, recompression is used primarily for the treatment of decompression sickness (DCS), arterial gas embolism and carbon monoxide poisoning. The shorter the time to instigation, the better the outcome. Recompression aims to increase oxygen solubility/delivery and nitrogen wash-out, decrease carbon monoxide concentration and gas bubble size, and reduce tissue ischaemia. DCS usually appears immediately on resurfacing, 98% within 24 hours. Delayed recompression after 48 hours still improves clinical outcome in the majority of cases. Pulmonary syndrome (chokes) in DCS occurs in around 2% of cases and can be fatal.

A6. (e). Decompression sickness results from mechanical effects of nitrogen bubbles. Osteonecrosis has been recorded in up to 50% of divers. Nitrogen enters and leaves fat tissue more slowly than oxygen or carbon dioxide.

A7. (d). Best fit. It typically affects large joints and is typically unaffected by movement. It can present 4 to 12 hours after exposure. The gas is dissolved in body tissues according to Henry's law.

A8. (a). Best fit. Blood is forced off the lower limbs and blood volume in the chest increases. Right atrial pressure can increase more than left. Ventilatory capacity can decrease. Resulting carbon dioxide retention and atrial naturetic hormone can be produced with a resultant diuresis.

Biological Hazards, Biological Monitoring and Vaccinations

A9. (b). SARS-CoV-2 (COVID-19) is an RNA virus. Spread is mostly by droplet transmission. There is no common association with adverse outcome in pregnancy. Fomite transmission is uncommon.

A10. (a). The risk of an individual developing serious or fatal COVID-19 depends on their personal vulnerability should infection occur. The female gender has a relative risk of 0.6. Non-white people have a relative risk ranging from 1.3 to 1.5. Body mass index greater than 30 but less than 35 kg/m^2 has a relative risk of 1.3. A notable feature of COVID-19 is that mortality rates increase exponentially with age. Smoking status does not carry any material increase in risk of an individual developing serious or fatal COVID-19.

A11. (e). Genetically modified organisms are not listed though their original wild species derivation may be listed. Group 1 is unlikely to cause human disease and a new agent should not be assumed to be in Group 1 initially. Group 3 causes severe disease but usually has available treatment and or vaccine. Advisory Committee on Dangerous Pathogens UK (ACDP) concerns itself with risks to humans.

A12. (d). Best fit. Over 60 pathogens, including viruses, have been reported as transmissible by NSIs. A systematic review showed a reduction in NSIs following legislation in two non-randomised studies considered to be of low-to-moderate quality. A meta-analysis showed that while safety engineered devices reduced injury rates by 49%, and education and training by 34%, the most effective intervention was a combination of both (62% reduction). Much of the current evidence in the area of NSI prevention is from studies at moderate and high risk of bias. The risk of hepatitis C is approximately 3% (1/30) or up to 10% if the source is RNA positive.

A13. (c). *Melitensis* is the most pathogenic and invasive species.

A14. (d). Anthrax is caused by the gram-positive bacteria *Bacillus anthracis*.

A15. (a). Lyme disease is caused by the spirochaete *Borrelia burgdorferi*, *Borrelia afzelii* and *Borrelia garinii*.

A16. (b). *Bacillus anthracis* spores have a long viability and as a result, pose a risk to workers who process animal hair, hides, bone products and wool.

A17. (a). Best fit. Standard Precautions are basic practices that are applied to the care of all patients regardless of the patient's suspected or confirmed infection status.

A18. (c). Best fit. Sharps safety is encompassed within Standard Precautions. Transmission-Based Precautions are practices that are implemented for the care of patients with documented or suspected infections where contact with the patient, their body fluids or their environment poses a risk, despite adherence to Standard Precautions. Contact, droplet and airborne precautions are the three elements of Transmission-Based Precautions.

A19. (d). Most common strain is *Salmonella typhimurium*.

A20. (c). A toxin is produced by the bacterium. Recovery is rapid (within six hours).

A21. (e). Found in human and animal excreta as well as on raw meat. Illness may last one to three days.

A22. (a).

A23. (b). Rare in the UK and Ireland. Anaerobic spore-producing bacterium which produces a potent toxin.

A24. (e). In general, bacteria do not multiply below 15°C and above 40°C. Spores will be killed only at high temperatures such as are found in boiling.

A25. (a). Most food poisoning outbreaks are the result of a food handler's poor hygiene.

A26. (b).

A27. (c). Non-return to work by those infected until shown to be clear of infection (stool sampling).

A28. (d). Also trained and informed staff. Good hygienic systems of work are important.

A29. (d). Rare in the UK. Imported bone/fish meal account for most cases. Hides, wool and hair from the Far and Middle East have potential to transmit the infection.

A30. (e). Occupations at risk include farmers, sewerage and watercourse workers.

A31. (a). Rare in the UK and Ireland. Occupational contraction is usually by handling infected animals (placental or foetal tissue in particular) or by inhalation of infected aerosols from such animals.

A32. (c).

A33. (b). Causes an atypical pneumonia.

A34. (c). HBeAg negative chronic HBV infection.

A35. (c). Best fit. A larger or additional vaccine dose may be required to induce protective antibodies in immunocompromised people. A titre of less than 10 mIU/ml is regarded as a non-responder after full vaccination and repeat course plus serology for previous infection. The HBeAg restrictions were removed by UKAP and viral load is the determining factor for EPPs. Hepatitis B vaccine can be given to the immunosuppressed though they may have a limited response. Through monitoring hepatitis B, seroconversions have been very rare. Non-responders can engage in EPPs but will need to comply with regular testing as per UKAP advice.

A36. (c). Best fit. UK NICE guidance indicates passengers should not be routinely contact traced. The IGRA test is a T-cell response. It is not the fact that evidence demonstrates ineffectiveness of BCG above 35 years of age, it is just that there is no research evidence of effectiveness above this age. Variably quoted but between 5% and 15% of latent TB converts to infection in a lifetime. At pre-placement there should also be enquiry about exposures and assessment of latent TB.

A37. (e). A patient with active TB may have a negative IGRA test result.

A38. (d). EPPs are procedures where there is a risk of injury to the healthcare worker (HCW) resulting in exposure of the patient's open tissues to the blood of the HCW. These procedures include those where the HCW's hands (whether gloved or not) may be in contact with sharp instruments, needle tips or sharp tissues (spicules of bone or teeth) inside a patient's open body cavity, wound or confined anatomical space where the hands or fingertips may not be always completely visible.

A39. (c). It does have incubation period of one to four weeks. Tetracyclines are the drug of choice. It is most frequently transmitted to humans by parrots. It is an infection caused by *Chlamydophilia psittaci*.

A40. (d). Best fit. A systematic review has shown that 18.7/100 healthcare workers have serologically proven influenza (often asymptomatic). Influenza vaccine is inactivated and is recommended in pregnancy. In a meta-analysis of randomised controlled trials, influenza vaccine was associated with a lower risk of major adverse cardiovascular events.

A41. (e). Best fit. Multiple analyses have shown an increased death rate attributable to pneumonia in welders, over many decades. Deaths were due to lobar, rather than broncho, pneumonia. Excess risk was also evident in other occupations exposed to metal fume (e.g., moulders, coremakers and furnace men in foundries). Inhalation of metal fume increases susceptibility to pneumonia, an effect which is reversed following cessation of exposure. An 'iron hypothesis' has been mooted to explain this whereby free iron can promote infection in bodily systems either as a nutrient for microorganisms or by damage to host cells from free radicals.

A42. (d). Best fit. Lyme disease is the only tick-borne disease in this list. It takes its name from Lyme, Connecticut, USA. It is an occupational zoonosis (i.e., an infectious disease transmitted from animals to humans and contracted in the course of employment). It is caused by bacterium *Borrelia burgdorferri* which is transmitted by the tick *Ixodes ricinus*. It is characterised by erythema chronicum migrans—an area of redness spreading out from the site of the bite. The tick is usually associated with deer. Neurological symptoms such as facial nerve neuritis, myelitis, encephalitis and meningitis may all occur as may a myocarditis. Chronic polyarthritis may also be found. Risk of contracting Lyme disease can be reduced by covering skin when outdoors, using insect repellent, inspecting clothes and body for ticks and having good personal hygiene.

A43. (a). Best fit. Hepatitis A vaccine is inactivated hepatitis A virus grown on diploid human cells and may be given in pregnancy if clinically indicated. It is also available in combination with hepatitis B. Inactivated quadrivalent flu vaccine contains two type A and two type B strains. Varicella vaccine is a live attenuated vaccine and is contraindicated in pregnancy. Even having completed a full course of tetanus vaccination (five doses), an adult's immunity may wane over time and boosters may be considered every 10 years.

A44. (d). Rapid degradation of mRNA within cells contributes to the safety profile of these vaccines.

A45. (c). Best fit. The lifetime risk of active TB when positive for latent TB is around 5% to 10%. It is true there is not much evidence for effectiveness of BCG after age 35 but prior to that the efficacy is less than 90%. In children it is usually quoted as 70% to 80% effective in preventing meningitis or miliary TB. Certificate evidence of BCG is a contraindication of further BCG. The 2020 report for England indicated nearly 50% of cases were pulmonary.

A46. (a). Urinary creatinine levels decrease with age in line with a reduction in the body's muscle mass. Biological monitoring, based on the analysis of hazardous substances or their metabolites in biological fluids, is a useful means of assessing systemic exposure through inhalation, ingestion and dermal absorption. The concentrations of analytes in urine collected by incomplete single voiding before, during or at the end of work, may be affected by urine concentration or dilution depending on the fluid balance. The most common approach to compensate for this involves measurement of the creatinine concentration in the sample and expression of the concentration of the analyte as a ratio of the creatinine concentration.

A47. (e). Biological monitoring (BM) remains useful in assessing the uptake of hexavalent chromium and control of exposure. Urine samples should be collected at the end of a work shift and analysed for total chromium. Care should be taken to ensure that any BM sampling is representative of the worker's typical workload. BM does not indicate exposure route (i.e., inhalation, ingestion or skin absorption), only that exposure has occurred.

A48. (b). Biological monitoring provides an indirect assessment of dermal exposure. Biological effect monitoring is a measurement of a biological effect in exposed workers. Biological monitoring is a surrogate of absorbed dose. It is not an example of primary prevention. Biological monitoring assists in evaluating if preventive measures are working.

A49. (c). All of the others are examples of biological monitoring.

A50. (b). Best fit. It can be performed by measuring blood toluene. Methyl hippuric acid is used for monitoring of xylene. It is not a form of biological effect monitoring and can be quite useful as toluene has a skin notation.

Environmental Protection

A51. (a). Smoking prevalence by workers varies according to industry. Workplace smoking bans have not been implemented globally. Thus, ETS continues to present an occupational hazard to the health of workers. Most large prospective cohort studies have found no link between breathing ETS and breast cancer. However, some case-control studies have shown a small increased risk, especially among premenopausal women.

A52. (e). No such correlation has been demonstrated. There is some suggestion that inadequate cleaning practices may contribute to symptoms and that thorough office cleaning may reduce symptoms. However, interventions to reduce dust (e.g., HEPA filters) have not been shown to reduce symptoms.

A53. (b). Lden reflects day, evening and night noise levels and best correlates with cardiovascular impacts. Lnight reflects night-time exposure only and would be most appropriate noise indicator for disturbance of sleep. LEX represents the measurement to reflect exposure during an 8-hour working day. LA,max is a useful indicator when particular noise events are being studied as it represents the maximum levels.

A54. (e). Electromagnetic field is measured in μT. Volt/metre is the unit for electric fields. The electric fields dropped to background levels of 52 at 100 m from the lines and IARC classify electromagnetic fields as being possibly carcinogenic.

A55. (a). Best fit. Some scientists suggest we are in a new geological era, not yet defined but characterised by the volume of made materials exceeding the volume of living beings for the first time in history. The Anthropocene has grown most rapidly in the 20th century, particularly since World War II. The precautionary principle is still controversial and lacks a definitive formulation with one view that uncertainty is not justification to delay the prevention of harm, whereas the other opines that no action (potentially causing harm) should be taken without certainty that no harm will result. While some definitions of endocrine disrupters (e.g., Webridge) encompass the term 'adverse' health effects, a more acceptable definition encompasses changes that 'may' lead to adverse or toxic effects after changes in endocrine function.

A56. (d). Best fit. An increased prevalence of serum biomarkers associated with later development of Barrett's oesophagus has been shown in the cohort of WTC-exposed FDNY firefighters with normal pre-9/11 lung function. This is not the case for the condition itself.

A57. (c). Best fit. It reflects that lack of scientific certainty, which is often the case in environmental assessments, should not be used to prevent otherwise positive actions.

Epidemiology and Statistics

A58. (c). The Bradford Hill criteria published in 1965, otherwise known as Hill's criteria for causation, are a group of nine principles that can be useful in establishing epidemiologic evidence of a causal relationship between a presumed cause and an observed effect and have been widely used in public health research.

A59. (c). Intention to treat is a pragmatic approach which reports on all those randomised to the study, regardless of whether they completed or disengaged for any reason (e.g., 'lost to follow-up'). It reflects what would happen in clinical practice. In a per protocol analysis, some randomised participants may later be excluded if they do not complete the protocol. Such an approach explores what might happen in ideal or experimental conditions.

A60. (e). First arrange the numbers in rank order as follows: 2, 3, 4, 7, 8, 8. The median is the average of the two middle observations, 4 and 7: 5.5.

A61. (d). A randomised controlled trial (or randomised control trial; RCT) is a type of scientific experiment (e.g., a clinical trial) or intervention study (as opposed to observational study) that aims to reduce certain sources of bias when testing the effectiveness of new treatments; this is accomplished by randomly allocating subjects to two or more groups, treating them differently and then comparing them with respect to a measured response.

A62. (e). Validity is an expression of the degree to which a test is capable of measuring what it is intended to measure. A study is valid if the results correspond to the truth.

A63. (a). An age-specific rate is the incidence or mortality rate for a specified age group in which the numerator and denominator refer to the same age group; it is expressed as the number of new cancer cases or deaths per 100,000 population at risk. Cancer incidence rates are strongly related to age for all cancers combined, with the highest incidence rates being in older people.

A64. (b). High sensitivity implies a low false negative rate.

A65. (e). A test is specific if there are few false positives.

A66. (d). This is a measure of the overall success of a test in correctly classifying subjects.

A67. (a).

A68. (c). Also known as reproducibility.

A69. (d). This is point prevalence and period prevalence. Prevalence rates are affected by the prognosis of a medical condition.

A70. (a). Refers to new cases only. Not affected by prognosis of a medical condition.

A71. (e). SMR is (O/E X 100) where O = number of observed deaths in a study population and E = the expected number of deaths. A value for an SMR greater than 100 indicates a higher number of deaths in the study group than expected.

A72. (c).

A73. (b). This measures the proportion of deaths in a cohort group and compares it with the proportion of deaths in the general population. A figure greater than 100 indicates a higher proportion of deaths in the cohort group.

A74. (b). The value of the mean can be influenced by a few isolated high or low values ('outliers').

A75. (a). Not widely used as may get a spurious result when the number of observations is small.

A76. (e). Not affected by outliers.

A77. (c).

A78. (d). Also known as a Gaussian distribution. Here the value of the mean, mode and median is the same.

A79. (d). One of the most widely used measures of variation. A low standard deviation implies high reproducibility.

A80. (a). A large value indicates the means are widely dispersed about the population mean.

A81. (e). The value ranges from +1 to –1. If it is positive this indicates both variables increase together.

A82. (c). Expressed as either 99% or 95% confidence intervals.

A83. (b).

A84. (c). The cohort study is the appropriate design to study incidence of a disease. Randomised controlled trials are interventional studies. Cross-sectional studies give an indication of prevalence. A case-control study cannot measure incidence because you start with cases and non-cases, so you cannot calculate relative risk.

A85. (c). Best fit. While 95% confidence intervals are appropriate in studying areas of interest or hypothesis they are not as helpful in looking at large numbers of hypothesis. A 95% CI suggests that there is a 1 in 20 chance of a finding being by chance alone. If in this case cancers are studied, by chance alone one would expect one or two of those to be in a statistically significant region. National cancer levels may be all that is available and may be more reliable than local levels.

A86. (e). The methods for the review, including how the quality of studies is assessed, should be agreed before the study commences, and should be published in the methods. The diamond represents the pooled results of the included studies. Clinical heterogeneity reflects varied methods such as selection of patients and range of interventions. Statistical heterogeneity reflects odds ratios amongst the studies—some indicate harm from the intervention, some benefit. It can be assessed using a Chi-squared test. A funnel plot is a graphical representation that illustrates whether there may be publication bias when selecting the studies for the analysis. A search strategy should include more than one database and include an adequate range of keywords and not just one language.

A87. (a). Best fit. All the responses are correct; however, the study must address the question it is attempting to answer as failure to do that renders everything else redundant. The article has to be relevant to the topic of interest, and it is essential to determine the quality of the study by assessing its appropriateness, including whether the study design was able to answer the hypothesis/research question.

A88. (b). 'I' refers to intervention, prognostic factor or exposure. In the first instance, PICO is an ideal starting point in addressing a research question. It provides a systematic framework from which to start a research project, regardless of whether the planned study is observational (case-control, systematic review) or interventional (randomised controlled trial of a drug or other treatment). It is therefore also useful in the critical appraisal of published research. In occupational health practice the population 'P' may be a group of exposed workers or be drawn from the general population or a subset thereof (e.g., pregnant women). 'I' refers to the intervention in the case of a therapeutic intervention but may be changed to 'E' (exposure) if the study is exploring historical workplace exposures (e.g., case-control study)—creating 'PECO'. 'C' refers to the comparison of one group to another and usually refers to a control group (e.g., receives no treatment or unexposed in the case of an occupational exposure study). 'O' refers to the outcome of the intervention (e.g., impact of treatment in placebo-controlled trial or disease outcome in the case of occupational exposure).

Fitness for Work, Rehabilitation and Shift Work

A89. (e). Vestibular rehabilitation therapy is the most effective treatment for continuous or chronic dizziness.

A90. (c). The other statements are 'red flags' which are possible indicators of serious spinal pathology.

A91. (a). HbA1c is a fraction of glycosylated haemoglobin (normal value less than 7%), and its measurement provides an accurate estimate of mean glucose levels over the preceding six weeks, which correlates with the risk of microvascular complications.

A92. (d). Loss of memory, learning difficulties and a decrease in the ability to concentrate on a task characterises cognitive impairment in the elderly. This ranges from mild deficits, which are not clinically detectable, to dementia at the severe end of the scale. There is some debate about the age-dependency ratio, but it has not stabilised. A compulsory retirement age is not impossible in the UK and Ireland, though employers would need to be very careful that they can demonstrate there is a legitimate aim and a compulsory retirement age is a proportionate means of achieving that aim. Those groups with higher levels of education tend to have better health in older age possibly linked to social circumstances and income. The healthy worker effect is relevant in the older worker given the higher rates of chronic disease that results in stopping work.

A93. (a). The recommended lighting is a Macbeth easel lamp, but daylight is a reasonable substitute. Should be viewed at arm's length. Delay of over four seconds suggests a mild deficit. Two errors on plates 2 to 13 of the 24-plate test indicate a red-green color deficit. Eyes are tested individually.

A94. (a). Subfertility has not been shown reliably but all the others have.

A95. (c). Nitrous oxide is classified as a pregnancy risk group Category C medication, meaning that there is a risk of foetal harm if administered during pregnancy. Chronic work-related exposure to high levels of nitrous oxide may cause increased risk of neurologic, renal and liver disease and increased risk of miscarriage and fertility issues among female dental assistants where 'scavenging equipment' is not used. The Public Health England study suggested the rate of reproductive disorder was closer to 30%. High-level carbon disulphide exposure will be directly toxic, but it is recognised that low-level chronic exposure can have an effect on male libido. Male semen and sperm quality can be affected by psychological stress. The Health, Safety and Welfare Regulations were introduced in 1992 in Great Britain.

A96. (c). Best fit. Iatrogenic vaginal clear cell adenocarcinoma occurred in young women exposed in utero to stilboestrol, an obstetric practice prevalent in some countries in the mid-20th century.

A97. (c). The Disabilities of the Arm, Shoulder and Hand (DASH) describes the disability experienced by people with upper limb disorders. A 10-point difference in DASH score may be considered as a minimal important change in functioning.

A98. (d). A higher QuickDASH score is associated with an unsuccessful RTW. Integrating mental healthcare provision with occupational rehabilitation is a potential programme approach to improve RTW.

A99. (e). Identifying negative perceptions may cause difficulties in the doctor–patient relationship and consequently, some doctors may choose to avoid this.

A100. (e). Work-related musculoskeletal disorders of the upper limb include a range of painful conditions involving muscles, tendons, joints and nerves. Interventions have been widely studied, but conclusions are hampered by both workplace and intervention heterogeneity leading to many low-quality studies. However, there is now strong evidence that resistance training can help prevent and manage symptoms while stress management training and EMG biofeedback have no impact (moderate evidence). Specific workstation additions have a role, but there is moderate to strong evidence that adjustment alone has no effect.

A101. (a). Best fit. Studies of COVID-19, MERS, SARS and Ebola outbreaks identified a range of protective factors (e.g., older experienced workers were less stressed as were those with less clinical contact and observing infected colleagues recover from illness) and helpful strategies (e.g., clear communication, training on infectious diseases, enforcement of infection control, adequate supplies of personal protective equipment and access to practical and psychological support). Increased levels of stress and psychological distress can persist for many months and in one study up to three years after the outbreak. The World Health Organization has published guidance on PFA which includes assessment of needs and dealing with basic needs (e.g., food and water).

A102. (c). Burnout interventions in healthcare have been widely reported and may be directed towards the individual or the work environment. Reviews of controlled interventions confirmed small but significant reductions in burnout following a range of individual and organisational interventions. Sub-group analysis confirmed small significant burnout reduction with individual physician interventions but medium significant reduction and larger effects with organisational interventions, supporting the view that burnout is likely to be a problem of organisations rather than individuals.

A103. (a). Financial compensation may initially appear to be a positive intervention; however, it is often an obstacle to successful rehabilitation.

A104. (b). In the absence of any other clinical signs such as the red flags mentioned in the question, this probably represents simple back pain and is best treated with core strengthening and normalisation of activity.

A105. (b). WHO define an impairment as 'any temporary or permanent loss or abnormality of a body structure or function, whether physiological or psychological. An impairment is a disturbance affecting functions that are essentially mental (memory, consciousness) or sensory, internal organs (heart, kidney), the head, the trunk or the limbs'.

A106. (c). Night workers are defined in EU Regulations as those who work between the hours of 12 midnight and 7:00 a.m.

A107. (d). Clockwise rotation of shifts is generally better tolerated. With modern diabetic control most diabetics can manage shift work. Fatigue, sleep disruption, mood disorder and gastrointestinal effects are the most common health issues for shift workers. Shift work sleep disorder typically occurs in 10–40% of shift workers.

A108. (a). The suprachiasmatic nucleus in the hypothalamus has a key role in regulating circadian rhythms. The neocortex is the largest part of the cerebral cortex and is the outermost layer that covers the structures of the brain.

A109. (a). Best fit. This may be partly due to greater social pressures on women for family and so forth. Older workers are more intolerant. Extraverts tolerate shift work better as do those with higher physical fitness. Diabetics have more potential health issues doing shift work.

A110. (b).

Best fit. Whilst all of the statements are correct, an RTW plan put together with the agreement of the employee, their manager and HR team is more likely to succeed. OH and Trade union representative can provide useful advice. Evidence confirms in those recovering from COVID-19 a proportion continue to experience symptoms such as fatigue, fever and cognitive dysfunction for weeks (5–36% of people) or even months (5–15% of people) after their infection. This has been called Long COVID Syndrome and impacts negatively on the individual's functioning both in regard to activities of daily living in addition to the ability to remain in or return to work.

Fumes, Mists, Dusts and Gases

A111. (c).

Metal fume fever is typically caused by exposure to zinc oxide fume. Tolerance develops over the working week, and onset is usually 4 to 12 hours after exposure. Symptoms dissipate spontaneously.

A112. (d).

Teflon is an accepted cause of polymer fume fever. Teflon flu is well recognised as a cause of fume fever and is a non-metal example of inhalation fever. Tachyphylaxis does tend to occur with continued exposure and symptoms present sometimes at the weekend when exposure stops. Onset times can vary but commonly quoted as between 4 and 10 hours.

A113. (c).

Best fit. Severity of coal worker's pneumoconiosis varies according to the composition of the coal. Simple coal worker's pneumoconiosis is not associated with an increased risk of lung cancer. Caplan syndrome is associated with rheumatoid arthritis. There has been a recent resurgence of PMF in US coal miners.

A114. (e).

Welder's disease. Siderosis results from exposure to iron ore and typically is associated with normal lung function and the finding of 'red lungs' at autopsy.

A115. (e).

Softwood dust comes from coniferous trees. Hardwood dust comes from deciduous trees. Associated with excess adenocarcinoma nasal cavity. Associated with anosmia.

A116. (d).

The CLP Regulation (for 'Classification, Labelling and Packaging') is a European Union regulation from 2008 aligning the EU system of classification, labelling and packaging of chemical substances and mixtures to the Globally Harmonised System (GHS). Ozone is too unstable to store and transport so does not come under the CLP Regulations. Ozone will attack and degrade rubber seals and gaskets and ozone levels tend to increase with temperature in populated areas.

A117. (c).

Ozone is typically a blueish colour and is pungent in high concentrations. Nitrogen dioxide is produced during the breakdown of silage in agriculture. Ozone is more soluble in inert non-polar solvents such as fluorocarbons.

A118. (c). CS2 is a solvent for oils and resins. Metabolites do appear in the urine. Biological monitoring is usually carried out after each shift. Mostly used in production of viscose rayon and cellophane.

A119. (d). Best fit. Carboxyhaemoglobin concentrations are typically less than 10% in smokers. Carbon monoxide results in the oxyhemoglobin dissociation curve shifting to the left impairing oxygen delivery to the tissues. Carbon monoxide is a by-product of incomplete combustion of carbon fuels. Carbon monoxide is generated in the human body by the catabolism of heme and results in the normal baseline human carboxyhemoglobin level of 0.4–1%.

A120. (d). Nitrogen, methane and carbon dioxide are 'simple' asphyxiants. Ammonia is an irritant gas. Carbon monoxide would be another example of a chemical asphyxiant.

A121. (e). Sulphur dioxide is a colourless gas released naturally by volcanic activity and is produced as a by-product of copper extraction and the burning of fossil fuels contaminated with sulphur compounds. The chemical formula is SO2. It is a toxic gas with the smell of burnt matches. It is soluble in water producing acid rain in the environment. Exposure is related to pre-term birth.

A122. (e). Hydrogen cyanide exposure results in an odour like that of bitter almonds. It interferes with aerobic metabolism resulting in lactic acidosis. Thiocyanate levels do not accurately reflect intensity of intoxication. HCn is a colourless gas above 25.6°C.

A123. (e). Best fit. While carbon monoxide exerts its toxic effect by binding to haemoglobin to produce carboxyhaemoglobin it also produces changes to the remaining haemoglobin which causes more avid binding of oxygen with a left shift in the oxygen dissociation curve. Chronic exposure is thought to accelerate atherogenesis and it may explain some of the vascular pathology seen in smokers. The medical significance of its binding to other haem containing proteins is unclear.

General OH Practice and Legal Issues

A124. (c). It will be retained in their health record which cannot be accessed without the employee's consent or a court order.

A125. (a). Tort is an act or omission that gives rise to injury or harm for which the courts impose liability.

A126. (c). All the others must exist, but breach of a statutory duty is not required but could be used as evidence in a claim.

A127. (b). Poor attendance may be a factor in a fair dismissal due to capability or frustration of contract but is not in itself considered a reason for a fair dismissal.

A128. (d). A detailed exposure assessment will be necessary only if a work-related disease is suspected. Then an in-depth history is needed of what the worker has been exposed to, for how long and in what quantities. The practice of occupational medicine is based on the concept of the effect of work on health and the effect of health on work. Hobbies and out-of-work activities may be relevant (e.g., the use of adhesives for model making in a case of occupational asthma). Previous job history is important, particularly if dealing with chronic disease. An accurate assessment will facilitate the provision of realistic and accurate advice to both employee and employers.

A129. (b). If the employee has persistent unsatisfactory work performance an underlying health condition may not prevent a dismissal taking place. However, established disciplinary procedures must have been followed and issues regarding disability, job adjustment and alternative work must also have been considered. Retirement on ill-health grounds could be an alternative option. Options for relocation and job change are also important considerations in keeping with relevant disability discrimination legislation that may be applicable.

A130. (b). Restrictions should have a good reason for being imposed and be based on sound health or safety grounds. Many disabled workers will be highly motivated to overcome their disability and hence attendance rates may be better than average. Provided they are correctly placed there is no increased safety risk. The occupational health team can give advice to an employer on modifications or adjustments needed to allow a disabled employee to be employed or remain in employment if the disability is progressive. Compliance with relevant disability discrimination legislation will have to be strictly always adhered to.

A131. (d). In many cases there may be no genuine medical illness present. This is more likely with short-term absence (fewer than 10 days) as against long-term absence. Certified sickness absence appears to increase with increasing age.

A132. (a). Pre-employment medicals are not a good tool for predicting sickness absence. Having a policy in place and working closely with the individual, their medical team and occupational health advisors will assist in the case management process. Any relevant disability discrimination legislation will have to be considered.

A133. (b). The role of the occupational health (OH) team should be divorced from the mechanics of any disciplinary procedures such as these. There will be a role for OH in taking samples as part of an agreed workplace alcohol (and drugs) policy. OH can also assist in supporting workers and facilitating abstinence programmes when available. Poor time-keeping, increased accident rates, abusive behaviour and overt smell of alcohol on breath at work are also indicators. In dealing with cases, medical confidentiality guidelines will apply.

A134. (d). Engaging with the workforce to get their support and buy-in is vitally important when planning a health promotion programme. All the other items listed are necessary for successful delivery.

A135. (e). Getting worker engagement is vital to securing their participation in a well-being programme. Offering general health promotion events is helpful, but without proper worker engagement the benefits to the organisation will be reduced. Programmes should be targeted, relevant and supportive.

A136. (d). This can be provided only with consent. In addition, an effective OH report will include details of any functional limitations or relevant disabilities that may temporarily or permanently affect the employee's ability to carry out their job. If the employee is absent, guidance in relation to the timescale for a return to full or restricted duties should be provided.

A137. (a). All of the above are useful inclusions in an OH report. Multiple sclerosis is a generally recognised disability. From the employer's perspective, the benchmark is whether the report assists them in their ongoing management of the case. This may include dealing with issues of disability, managing a return to work or ongoing absence or preparing for termination of employment on health grounds. The OH practitioner should be assisting the employer by providing timely, relevant and appropriate reports. It is important to ensure that the employee understands the process in which they are engaged and that written informed consent for a report to be prepared has been obtained. It would also be good practice to inform the employee at the conclusion of a consultation what the report is likely to contain. Under UK guidelines the employee should be offered a copy of the report for their agreement or otherwise in advance of it being sent to the employer.

A138. (b). Handling of information, including with whom it is stored and shared, is of paramount importance when a report is being prepared on an employee. Written consent from the employee is always advised. There will be limited occasions when the public interest or a legal duty applies whereby consent is not required. Many jurisdictions will have data protection regulations that need to be complied with.

A139. (c). An assessment should not be undertaken without either oral or preferably written consent of the employee. It is good practice to explain the content of the report to the employee and offer a copy should the employee wish to have one.

A140. (a). Staff number would already be available to the employer and unlikely to be considered sensitive personal data. The employee's medical diagnosis and treatment are considered highly sensitive data. In addition the employee's date of birth and telephone number are also considered sensitive.

A141. (e). Best fit. Opinion in a report is advice only. There may be conflicting advice from other sources such as the general practitioner in which case the employer is free to choose which advice they follow, though they may need to be prepared to justify their choice later. The assessor should check the details of the referral were discussed and read out the referral to the employee if there is any confusion. The point of view of the employee should be considered. Opinion based on an error of fact would be subject to change; otherwise, there is not an expectation to alter an opinion. In some cases, one may create an addition that identifies the employee's view is different on an issue. The employee can withdraw their consent at any stage. In practical terms once the report has been sent to the employer it is difficult to change the situation. Functional details give an idea of what the employee can still do, and this can be compared with the limitations of the medical problems they have and the tasks they may need to perform in work.

A142. (e). While it is good practice to ensure that the consent is documented in writing, it is not an essential part of informed consent. Informed consent should always be documented whether it is in writing or verbal.

A143. (b). While these would all be considered standard elements of a referral, there are additional requirements that will inform a quality report. The referral letter should include specific questions to be addressed in the report (e.g., fitness for work, likely date of return to work if absent, the need for any adjustments, details of any relevant workplace incident, for example injury, the impact of health on work and the context in relation to any ongoing issues, for example pending disciplinary action). All things considered, a good quality referral will generate a good quality report.

Health Surveillance

A144. (e). Risk assessment should be used to identify any need for health surveillance. Health surveillance should not be a substitute for undertaking a risk assessment or using effective controls.

A145. (c). Body Mass Index Measurement Programme. Health surveillance is a scheme of repeated health checks which are used to identify ill health caused by work.

A146. (a). Health surveillance does not minimise or eliminate exposure to hazards. Health surveillance is important for highlighting lapses in workplace control measures, therefore providing invaluable feedback to the risk assessment.

A147. (a). Best fit. Health surveillance should be introduced only after all other controls (within the hierarchy of controls) have been implemented and risk assessment confirms an ongoing risk to human health for which health surveillance will provide additional protection. Anonymised group results should be fed back to staff and health and safety committees. Personally identified data should be disclosed only to the individual concerned unless consent to further release is given. Periodic skin inspection of 'at-risk' staff by a 'responsible person' is more appropriate than an annual questionnaire and for certain hazards, only an approved medical practitioner can supervise this role (e.g., vinyl chloride). All workers exposed to the hazard should be included in health surveillance, regardless of whether baseline data are available.

A148. (a). Biological monitoring is measuring exposure and not health effects so is not health surveillance.

A149. (d). Best fit. Health surveillance should be based on the actual risks as opposed to hazards. The SDS may show hazards but are relevant only when one knows whether there is actual exposure to levels that may cause harm.

A150. (a). Spirometry can be performed, if necessary, as early as seven days after an uncomplicated MI. Spirometry should be deferred in the case of an acute illness that may precipitate vomiting. Forced expiration may aggravate the other conditions.

A151. (c). Most audiometers use a modified Hughson–Westlake method. It can show a unilateral loss but further tests such as an MRI are required to diagnose acoustic neuromas. A clinical assessment is required to help differentiate conductive from sensorineural loss. It can be performed in a quiet room if it meets the ISO standard. If noise levels exceed relevant action levels audiometry is required even if personal protective equipment is worn.

A152. (c). Unit of measurement is lux which is lumen per square metre.

A153. (a). Unit of measurement is candela.

A154. (e). Unit of measurement is candela per square metre.

A155. (b). Usually expressed as a light reflectance value (LRV).

A156. (d). Unit of measurement is lumen.

Mental Health, Psychosocial Work Environment and Stress

A157. (a). Maslow's Hierarchy of Needs includes these five levels that allow an individual to feel fulfilled. It is often applied to the workplace to determine how to motivate employees and make sure their needs are met more effectively.

A158. (b). Employees who are obese are also at an increased risk for presenteeism.

A159. (e). Best fit. The model incorporates Positive Emotion, Engagement, Relationships, Meaning and Accomplishment. Martin Seligman and others began to shift the research focus from mental illness and pathology to studying what is positive; thus began the Positive Psychology movement in the late 1990s. Working on aspects of PERMA not only improves well-being but also decreases psychological distress. PERMA incorporates both eudaimonic and hedonic components, setting well-being theory apart from other theories of well-being.

A160. (b). Fluoxetine is an SSRI, and these have been found to improve PTSD (statistically significant).

A161. (d). Psychologically focused debriefing is not useful in either the prevention or treatment of PTSD. Cognitive processing therapy and prolonged exposure therapy are approved trauma-focused treatment interventions in adults (NICE Guidelines 2019). EMDR should be considered when trauma is non-combat-related. EMDR should be provided by trained practitioners with ongoing supervision.

A162. (a). The UK Health and Safety Executive launched the management standards that offers a step-by-step approach to the assessment and management of the causes of work-related stress. These standards define the characteristics and culture of an organisation where work-related stress is being managed effectively and provide a benchmark by which an organisation can measure their performance. They include seven work areas that cover the primary sources of stressors at work. The other work areas that cover the primary sources of stressors at work include Relationships and Demands.

A163. (c). Personality disorders are relatively common but are not easily diagnosed and require a structured clinical assessment process. There is no single approach to treating personality disorders. Talking therapies can be used and include cognitive behavioural therapy (CBT), dialectical behaviour therapy (DBT), cognitive analytical therapy (CAT) and psychodynamic/ psychoanalytic therapy. Medication may include anti-depressants; mood stabilisers; anti-psychotic medications and anxiolytics. Substance abuse is not uncommon in personality disorder but is probably less than 20%, not 50%. Those diagnosed with a personality disorder have been recognised as having a disability as defined in EU/UK disability discrimination legislation.

A164. (d). Best fit. Burnout, first described by Freudenberger in 1974, has now been added to the International Classification of Diseases and is characterised by three dimensions. It is conceptualised as resulting from chronic workplace stress which has not been managed. Burnout shares features of depression (hopelessness, poor self-esteem) but requires intervention at workplace level.

A165. (b). The management standards derive largely from the DCS (demand, control, support) model of workplaces stress informed by the work of Karasek, who proposed the theory in 1979 and expanded upon it in cooperation with Theorell in 1990. The Standards also incorporate the areas of role, relationships and change.

A166. (d). Best fit. Studies are largely cross-sectional with self-report surveys and further research is needed to establish a causal link. There are many aspects to job control, including objective versus perceived control and locus of control which is different from self-efficacy. A meta-analysis shows the relationship between perceived control and locus of control to be modest. The relationship between control and stress can be confounded by additional variables, with varying degrees of correlation which may be statistically significant but weak. The allostatic load model of stress does not incorporate the measurement of control.

A167. (a). Best fit. Organisational justice (OJ) has emerged as a model of occupational stress which can explain deleterious health effects. It refers to perceived equity in the social norms governing companies. It incorporates distributive justice (how benefits are distributed), procedural justice (the policies and procedures governing that distribution) and interactional justice (or interpersonal relationships) which itself can be subdivided into relational (respect received from management) and informational (explanations about new procedures) justice. A systematic review of prospective studies has confirmed that while controlling for demand/control/support and effort–reward imbalance, relational justice had a significant effect on mental health and sickness absence. It was also the most frequently measured component of OJ. Procedural justice was a strong predictor of self-rated health and of minor psychiatric morbidity.

A168. (d). All the others are components of the UK Health and Safety Executive Management Standards approach to workplace stress.

A169. (e). Best fit. The ERI posits that a lack of reciprocity between the effort of work and the rewards gained leads to strain. These are the model's extrinsic components. High effort and low reward indicate a reciprocity deficit which is hypothesised to lead to strong negative emotions leading to sustained autonomic and endocrine activation and negative health outcomes. Certain personality characteristics aggravate the imbalance, including the coping pattern of over-commitment (the intrinsic component) but may have a direct rather than moderating effect. Effort resembles demand in the P-E fit model, whereas reward is closely linked with supplies so the ERI model can be seen as embedded in the former model.

A170. (d). Best fit. People who experience SSDs present with a preoccupation with and an unconscious exaggeration of physical symptoms. CBT may relieve symptoms with therapy focused on distorted thoughts, unrealistic beliefs and behaviours that feed the anxiety. In relation to workplace injuries it can transform excessive stress into an acceptable form of disability.

A171. (c). Best fit. The American Psychiatric Association Diagnostic and Statistical Manual of Mental Disorders *(DSM-5)* states that post-traumatic stress disorder requires the victim to experience intense horror, fear or helplessness in the life-threatening instant and any allegedly traumatic event that does not meet this criterion must be discounted.

A172. (d). Staff who do not turn up to work should be contacted as their non-attendance may be indicative of poor mental health. Mental health support is particularly important for those who are seriously or persistently distressed. Managers should pay particular attention to HCWs in high-risk groups, such as those with a BAME (Black, Asian, and Minority Ethnic) background, and junior or inexperienced staff who have been working above their expected level of competence. Anyone who has been exposed to a potentially traumatic event should be actively monitored, particularly those considered at higher risk of developing mental health problems. Given the likelihood that HCWs have been exposed to morally distressing circumstances during the COVID-19 pandemic, most probably repeatedly, managers should help them to make sense of their experiences.

Musculoskeletal Disorders and Ergonomics

A173. (e). Frozen shoulders typically resolve in 12 to 18 months.

A174. (c). Gait disturbance is a red flag. An appropriate history and physical examination directed towards uncovering signs that suggest a serious underlying cause of low back pain is very important. Red flags also include pain that lasts more than six weeks, pain in persons younger than 18 years or older than 50 years, pain that radiates below the knee, a history of major trauma, constitutional symptoms, atypical pain (e.g., that which occurs at night or that is unrelenting), the presence of a severe or rapidly progressive neurological deficit, urinary and/or faecal incontinence, poor rectal tone and a history of malignancy.

A175. (a). Fear avoidance behaviour is a yellow flag. Weight loss is a red flag; litigation is a black flag; poor job satisfaction, fear of reinjury and fear of movement are also yellow flags.

A176. (a). There is no indication for electrophysiological studies unless the clinical picture is suggestive of nerve entrapment. Pathophysiology is uncertain and while ergonomics (in work and elsewhere) play a part, psychosocial risk factors are also important. It is important to rule out cervical pathology in any upper limb presentation.

A177. (d). The 'scarf test' is useful in confirming pathology of the acromioclavicular joint. The 'empty can' test assesses the function of the supraspinatus muscle. Phalen's manoeuvre is useful in carpal tunnel syndrome and Gerber's lift-off test assesses the subscapularis.

A178. (c). Typical features are median nerve distribution of tingling and pain, being woken at night by hand symptoms such as pain or numbness, pains in the wrist radiating into the forearm, median nerve distribution of blunting of sensation, positive Tinel and Phalen's tests. It is noted that the Mills test is used in assessing epicondylitis.

A179. (a). In most cases, the lesion involves the specialised junctional at the origin of the common extensor muscle at the lateral humeral epicondyle, specifically the tendinous origin of the extensor carpi radialis brevis (ECRB), and in 35% of the cases, the origin of the extensor carpi radialis longus (ECRL) will also be overstrained.

A180. (c). Affects 1–3% of adults annually. More commonly in dominant arm. Most common between ages of 35 and 50 years old. Men and women equally affected. The diagnosis is primarily a clinical one.

A181. (c). DD is associated with smoking. DD is a benign fibroproliferative disease affecting the palmar and digital aponeurosis. In later stages, it is characterised by the chronic contracture of the fourth and/or fifth finger of the hand towards the palm and is usually accompanied by a thickening of the palmar skin. These clinical manifestations significantly impair and restrict hand functioning.

A182. (c). There is an absence of a reliable evidence base linking CTS to vibrating tools or keyboard work. Twin studies indicate that genetic factors may account for up to half of cases in females. Compression of the median nerve in the carpal tunnel results in symptoms.

A183. (a). All the rest are black flags, which are system or contextual obstacles.

A184. (d). Tinel's is surprisingly poorly sensitive. Phalen's is somewhat more so but less that the carpal compression test, which applies pressure over the carpal tunnel for 30 seconds. Finkelstein's tests for de Quervain's tenosynovitis.

A185. (d). There is a significant body of evidence that application of the classically taught distribution of symptoms from CTS may be applying inappropriate diagnostic constraint. There should be a low threshold for nerve conduction studies to rule CTS in or out.

A186. (c). Best fit. There is insufficient evidence to state whether split keyboards are effective in reducing symptoms. The evidence for the positive impact of tracker ball devices is limited. There is moderate evidence that forearm supports have a positive impact on UEMSDs. The evidence for the benefit of a tactile feedback signal on the computer mouse (to reduce tension in extensor forearm muscles) is moderate and based on three studies, including two of high quality. There seems to be no effect from a joystick pointing device, albeit based on limited evidence.

A187. (e). The most common cause of these symptoms if chair being set too low in relation to keyboard/mouse height. This leads to subconscious raising shoulder and abduction of elbows. The chair height should allow shoulders to be relaxed and elbows to be beside the body.

A188. (b). Best fit. A job analysis will assess the tasks being carried out and hence highlight the hazards present and the exposure of the worker to those hazards. All of the other statements are correct. In regard to annual health surveillance, whilst this is not a requirement under COSHH regulations, there is some evidence for assessing workers as part of the risk assessment process for the presence of personal risk factors and early detection of physical symptoms.

A189. (d). The screen height should be lower for users of bifocal lenses as they tend to look at the screen through the bottom half of the lens. Screen height should be between 0 and 30 degrees below eye level for most users. The most important determinant of head posture is the position of the visual target hence the importance of screen height.

Noise, Vibration and Thermal Environment

A190. (d). Given that there are 10 dB between each of the three noise levels, this means that there is 10 times more noise energy at 92 dB than at 82 dB which is 10 times again 72 dB. The easiest way to make the estimate is to use the equal energy principal. By far and away the more significant contribution to the day is the one hour at 92 dB. That equates to two hours at 89 dB, by taking 3 dB and doubling the time. This also equates to four hours at 86 dB by again taking 3 dB away and doubling the time. The four hours at 72 dB contribute relatively little to the overall dose so can be ignored for the assessment. The daily exposure therefore can be simplified as equating to four hours at 86 dB and three hours at 82 dB. Clearly the average noise exposure must therefore be above 82 dB but below 86 dB. Hence, 84 dB is the only given answer which meets this criterion.

A191. (d). Best fit. Hearing protection is compulsory once the noise level is above the upper action level but in a designated hearing protection zone the hearing protection should be worn even in areas within the zone that are between the upper and lower action levels.

A192. (b). Best fit. Hearing-impaired listeners make significantly more consonant errors than normal hearing listeners both in quiet and in presence of background noise. With hearing impairment, the first thing to go is the ability to clearly hear high-pitched sounds especially in situations where there's considerable background noise. Typically 3 dB is quoted as doubling the sound energy in the UK. The A-weighted equivalent is closer to 40 dB. The 4 kHz region in the cochlea is further along and there remains debate as to all the factors for the 4 kHz notch.

A193. (c). Age-related hearing loss or presbycusis results in gradual deterioration of hearing, commencing in the higher frequencies and typically there is no notch.

A194. (a). A-weighting mimics the response of the human ear. C-weighting is used when measuring peak sound pressure. Are not measured in audiometry. In A-weighting the decibel values of sounds at low frequencies are reduced, compared with unweighted decibels.

A195. (c). Good correlation between dB(A) levels and risk of noise-induced deafness and annoyance of noise.

A196. (d). Is used to represent personal exposure over an 8-hour period. Also known as Leq(8h) and Lex(8h).

A197. (e). Lep'd of 90 dB(A). The level to which noise levels should, if possible, be reduced below.

A198. (a). Can be used to calculate Lep'd.

A199. (b). A sudden very loud or impact noise.

A200. (b). Best fit. Workers exposed to tools with a dominant frequency in the range of 60–300 Hz are more likely to develop the symptoms of HAVS. In contrast, workers using hand tools that emit a lower dominant frequency (i.e., 10–60 Hz) can display symptoms of HAVS. However, the tools with a lower dominant frequency are more likely to induce a loss of muscle mass and joint injuries in the elbow and shoulder. It is categorised using the Stockholm Workshop Scale. It is typically somewhat asymmetrical which is why each hand is scaled separately. It can improve on removal from vibration although not always.

A201. (b). Jobe's test is a physical exam test that is used to detect anterior shoulder instability. It is used to distinguish between anterior instability and primary shoulder impingement. Allen's test is used to assess the arterial blood supply of the hand. Phalen's manoeuvre is a provocative test used in the diagnosis of carpal tunnel syndrome. Roos stress test is used in the identification of thoracic outlet syndrome. Finkelstein's test is used to diagnose de Quervain's tenosynovitis in people who have wrist pain.

A202. (d). Best fit. The early signs and symptoms of HAVS are tingling and numbness in the fingers (which can cause sleep disturbance); loss of feeling in the fingers; loss of strength in your hands (you may be less able to pick up or hold heavy objects); in cold and wet conditions, the tips of the fingers go white then red and are painful on recovery (vibration white finger). Tingling that lasts 20 minutes or more after vibrating tool use is regarded as significant in HAVS assessment. Tingling that lasts 10 minutes is less likely to be vibration related. Specialised testing of vibration and temperature sensation thresholds is not a routine part of assessment. CTS can cause thumb sensory symptoms a history of smoking is relevant to the vascular component of HAVS and the differential cause of the hand symptoms. Those at risk are those who regularly use hand-held or hand-guided power tools and machines.

A203. (d). WBV is associated with road surface and speed and poor vehicle suspension. Cold environments are a risk factor for vibration white finger. WBV typically associated with increased bone mass.

A204. (b). Stage 0 is no attacks. Stage 1 is occasional attacks affecting the tips of one or more fingers. Stage 4 involves trophic skin changes in the fingertips. Objective evidence of vascular obstruction is usually not required.

A205. (e). Best fit. Low intensity exposure can be tolerated for longer periods then high intensity exposure. Visual performance is impaired in the range of 10 to 25 Hz. Vertical vibration is generally more harmful than horizontal vibration for seated workers. Vibration effect does depend on the frequency of vibration as well as acceleration, duration and direction.

A206. (c). Best fit. With a doubling of risk in pooled estimates having been shown in a systematic review. Causality has not been established between low back pain and WBV in farmers. The occupational link between WBV and hospitalisation has been suggested in a Swedish cohort study but requires further exploration. Observational studies have suggested links between prostate cancer and WBV but significant increase in risk has not been demonstrated to date. Significant improvements in bone mineral density of femoral neck have been shown in postmenopausal women exposed to training involving WBV.

A207. (e). Best fit. While all have been linked to whole-body vibration the evidence for most is quite weak. Strongest association is for simple low back pain.

A208. (c). Transmission is associated with metal surfaces, along with the following: low air exchange rates, insufficient distancing between workers, poor compliance with face mask use, presenteeism because of insecure poorly paid employment, limited or non-existent hygiene measures and overcrowded domestic accommodation for migrant workers.

A209. (d). WBGT is a measure of the heat stress in direct sunlight, which considers temperature, humidity, wind speed, sun angle and cloud cover (solar radiation). This differs from the heat index, which takes into consideration temperature and humidity and is calculated for shady areas.

A210. (d). Excessive sweating with clammy skin is a sign. Lack of sweating suggests heat stroke.

A211. (c). Some medications, most commonly antihistamines (taken for allergies), diuretics (taken for high blood pressure or leg swelling), laxatives (taken to relieve constipation), calcium channel blockers (one type of blood pressure or heart medicine), medicines for Parkinson's disease, some diarrhoea treatments, and tricyclic anti-depressants. SSRIs (Selective Serotonin Reuptake Inhibitors) can reduce serum sodium which decreases thirst and this could lead to accelerated dehydration during extreme heat conditions.

A212. (c). Symptoms of hypothermia can vary depending on how long someone has been exposed to the cold temperatures. Early symptoms: shivering, fatigue, loss of coordination, confusion, disorientation. Late symptoms: no shivering, blue skin, dilated pupils, slow pulse and breathing, loss of consciousness.

A213. (b). The core body temperature is greater than 40°C.

A214. (b). The absence of shivering can be an indicator of the seriousness of the condition.

A215. (c). Surface area is also important.

A216. (d).

A217. (a). Depends on the difference between temperature of skin or clothing and the surrounding surfaces (e.g., walls, machinery).

A218. (e).

A219. (b). This index gives a measure of the warmth of the environment.

Occupational Cancer

A220. (d). It is a Group 2A carcinogen (probably carcinogenic to humans). Ethanol and formaldehyde are both Group 1 carcinogens causing liver and gastrointestinal/haematopoietic malignancy respectively and ethylene oxide (breast cancer and lymphoid tumours). PCB have been upgraded from Group 2A to Group 1 by IARC (melanoma).

A221. (d). This is a Group 2B carcinogen with all the others classified as Group 1.

A222. (a). ICOH Statement on Occupational Health New Avenues for Prevention of Occupational Cancer and Other Severe Occupational Health Hazards; Dublin 2018.

A223. (d). The most common occupational cause is vinyl chloride monomer but not PVC which is the end-product or the other substances.

A224. (c). All the others are associated with increased risk of occupational cancer.

A225. (b). Cancer screening involves looking for cancer before symptoms appear when cancer may be easier to treat. As such it is not a primary preventive measure such as stopping smoking.

A226. (c). Best fit. Myeloid leukaemias in general are more commonly linked to occupational exposures.

A227. (d). Best fit. Night shift work is classified as 2A, a 'probable' human carcinogen.

A228. (c). Sunlight is important to those who work regularly outdoors such as roadworkers and farmers. Also ionising radiation.

A229. (a). Examples are benzidine and MOCA. Chemical, dyestuff, rubber cable industries.

A230. (b). VCM is associated with angiosarcoma of the liver.

A231. (e). Also, arsenic trioxide and arsenites found in smelting and pesticides. There is an increased risk of lung cancer in asbestos-exposed workers who smoke.

A232. (d). A rare adenocarcinoma. The very fine dust produced by power tools on hardwoods is particularly carcinogenic.

Occupational Hygiene

A233. (e). The Ames test, which is an in-vitro test for mutagenesis, utilises Salmonella typhimurium strain which is histidine-dependent and is grown on a histidine-deficient agar. This makes it an auxotrophic strain.

A234. (a). Face velocity is the air velocity at the opening of a hood. Transport velocity is the minimum velocity required to keep collected particles airborne in a system. Total pressure is the sum of static and velocity pressures at a point in an airstream. A smoke test gives an overall view of performance but does not allow for quantification.

A235. (a). The dermal uptake of a chemical is estimated by the permeability coefficient, the concentration of the substance on the skin, the area of skin exposed and the duration of exposure.

A236. (e). The requirement for health surveillance is dependent on the level of residual risk. It is not always required when there is exposure to asthma-causing agents if there is no residual risk after the control measures are in place. Health surveillance may be required even when exposures are below the occupational exposure limits. It differs from medical screening which is typically related to health promotion and generally does not distinguish between the health effects of exposure and those from pre-existing conditions.

A237. (d). Carbon monoxide is a gas, and benzene can emit vapours but not fumes. Fumes are typically less than 1 μm. They are formed by evaporation from melting metal but are relatively short lived. They will often react with airborne oxygen to form a metal oxide and may aggregate to form dusts.

A238. (d). Movements of air with outside wind is the wind pressure effect. The stack effect occurs in buildings when the outdoor temperature is substantially colder than the inside temperature. Lighter hot air rises, so the warmer, indoor air is buoyant and moves upward to exit the building through a variety of openings in the upper floors whilst cooler air is drawn in through gaps in the building structure.

A239. (c). Modern sampling pumps come with a wide range of capabilities and can usually be adjusted depending on the requirements of the sampling. Low-flow pumps are typically 1 ml to 200 ml per minute. Standard flow pumps are typically 0.5 L to 3 L per minute and high-flow problems are typically 3 L to 30 L per minute.

A240. (a). The lumen is the SI-derived unit of luminous flux, a measure of the total quantity of visible light emitted by a source per unit of time. Lumens are related to lux in that one lux is one lumen per square metre. The candela is the base unit of luminous intensity, that is, luminous power per unit solid angle emitted by a point light source in a particular direction.

A241. (e). The essential steps involve anticipation, recognition, evaluation and control of the hazard.

A242. (a).

A243. (d).

A244. (c). Previously known as TLVs. Represent a level to which an employee can be exposed without harming their health. There are two types of OES: an OEL (occupational exposure limit) and an MEL (maximal exposure limit).

A245. (b). OEL can be long term (i.e., over an 8-hour period), expressed as a time-weighted average (TWA) or short term (STEL), usually 10 minutes.

A246. (d). This is a detector tube that contains a chemical reagent which produces a colour change when a contaminated air sample is drawn through it.

A247. (e). This is a liquid-filled thermometer with a large, silvered bulb and a smaller bulb. It measures the cooling power of air, and using a formula the air velocity can be calculated.

A248. (a). Contains a wet and dry bulb—the difference in readings is used to calculate the humidity of air.

A249. (b). Usually used to monitor levels of dust or vapour in the worker's breathing zone.

A250. (c).

A251. (c). Decibel is a measure of sound intensity expressed on a logarithmic scale.

A252. (a).

A253. (b).

A254. (e).

A255. (d). The Sievert is an expression of the dose equivalent and is an index of the risk of harm following exposure to ionising radiation.

A256. (d). Best fit. Toluene and xylene are toxicological similar and synergistic, and they are considered additive. The effective measurement is therefore 110% of the OEL. Biological monitoring may be valuable but will not change the inadequate control situation.

A257. (c). Asbestos exposure is most associated with removal of lagging and insulation. Silica exposure is associated with an excess of tuberculosis. There is a synergistic effect with smoking rather than additive. Crocidolite is an amphibole asbestos.

A258. (e). Nanoparticles are usually defined in the range of 1 nm to 100 nm. 1 μm is 1,000 nm. Dust emission from construction is usually larger. High levels of PM1 have been linked with both respiratory and cardiovascular mortality—one of the reasons why diabetics are at high risk. WHO has AQG for PM10 and PM2.5 but not PM1.

A259. (e). PAP is one possible adverse health effect of silica exposure in addition to silicosis and lung cancer. Although PAP is a rare pulmonary disease, it should be considered when patients exposed to silica dust complain of chest tightness and cough and when there are typical signs of PAP radiologically.

A260. (d). Best fit. The health effects of nanoparticles are not fully understood. This makes it difficult to determine the risk with certainty and therefore how to mitigate these risks in the context of exposure. Risk assessment for exposure is a primary procedure. REACH definition is 1 nm to 100 nm as a dimension. HARNs high aspect ratio nanoparticles usually have a ratio of 1:3 or greater. There does remain concern about the health effects of graphene nanotubes and ratio can exceed 1:4. Health effects are not thought to be related to insolubility and most are soluble.

Radiation: Ionising and Non-Ionising

A261. (c). Radiation protection is governed by the principle of ALARA (as low as reasonably achievable). These are the limits for classified workers (known as Category A in the EU). Hospital workers would usually fall into Category B (non-classified), and limits for this group (option 'd') are substantially lower than for Category A workers.

A262. (b). Best fit. In radiation protection, most adverse health effects of radiation exposure can be divided into two broad classes whereby deterministic effects are threshold effects directly related to the absorbed dose of radiation (with increased severity as dose increases) in contrast to stochastic (non-deterministic) effects which occur by chance and generally do not require a threshold. The probability of stochastic effects occurring is increased with an increasing dose.

A263. (d). Stochastic effects such as induction of cancer and genetic defects are probabilistic events and may differ among individuals. The linear no-threshold hypothesis emphasises the stochastic nature of DNA damage caused by ionising radiation.

A264. (d). Radon will come under the Ionising Radiation Regulations 2017. While Scotland does have some areas of elevated radon levels, southwest of England and Wales and west of Northern Ireland have the areas of highest concentration. Radon is relevant to domestic and workplaces and has no odour. The significant risk is lung cancer.

A265. (c). Angiocardiogram to determine heart function (6,000 μSv). Dental X-ray (10 μSv). Chest X-ray (20 μSv). Mammography to identify breast cancer (500 μSv). CT scan (5,400 μSv).

A266. (e). Radon. On average, a person receives 1,995 μSv per year from radon in the home and an additional 229 μSv from radon in the workplace. On average, a person receives 350 μSv every year from thoron. On average, a person receives 302 μSv every year from cosmic radiation exposure. On average, a person receives 295 μSv every year from natural radioactivity in soils. On average, a person receives 262 μSv every year from natural radioactivity in food.

A267. (b). Stochastic effects occur by statistical chance.

A268. (d). Stochastic health effects are assumed not to have a threshold dose below which they do not occur. This is the reason that no level of radiation dose is considered to be completely 'safe' and why doses should always be kept as low as reasonably achievable (ALARA).

A269. (c). Neutron particles are high-speed nuclear particles that are the only type of ionising radiation that can make objects radioactive.

A270. (a). Alpha particles cannot penetrate most other materials. A piece of paper, the dead outer layers of skin or even a few inches of air are sufficient to stop alpha particles. Radioactive material that emits alpha particles can be very harmful to living cells when alpha particles are inhaled, ingested or absorbed into the blood stream (e.g., through a cut in or area of non-intact skin).

A271. (c). Neutrons have an exceptional ability to penetrate materials. Hydrogen-containing materials (concrete or water) are best for shielding neutrons.

A272. (a). IR dose limits are recommended by the International Commission on Radiation Protection, aim to prevent non-stochastic effects, and limit stochastic effects. A controlled area is one which has been designated by an employer to assist in controlling and restricting radiation exposures where the employer has recognised the need for people entering the area to follow special procedures.

A273. (a). Film badges are more sensitive to heat and humidity but can be retained as a permanent record unlike TLD information. The risk assessment includes any use of personal protective equipment.

A274. (e). Two types, electrons with a negative charge and positrons with a positive charge. They pose a problem to skin and subcutaneous tissues and to internal organs if ingested or inhaled into the body.

A275. (c). Decay means the unstable nature of certain atomic nuclei-emitting charged particles, electromagnetic waves or neutrons to allow adoption of a more stable state.

A276. (d).

A277. (b). Are a form of electromagnetic radiation.

A278. (a). Are positively charged. Have difficulty penetrating the dead outer layer of skin. Do not represent a significant hazard unless absorbed into the body (e.g., by ingestion, inhalation, wound contamination).

A279. (b). Beta particles, essentially electrons, cause ionising radiation.

A280. (d). Luminous intensity is measured in candela. Illuminance units are lumens per square metre. Luminous intensity is the term applied to luminous flux emitted per solid angle. Luminance is measured in candela per square metre. Brightness is a subjective attribute of light.

A281. (c). Occupational photokeratitis typically results from exposure to UV light such as welding, known as arc eye, and results in temporary damage to the cornea.

A282. (d). Best fit. Radio frequency radiation is part of the electromagnetic radiation spectrum incorporating microwaves. Frequency is measured in Hertz. RF radiation can cause thermal injury but does not ionise tissues. The risk of thermal injury increases with higher intensities of radiation and closer proximity, but other factors (including environmental humidity) can also contribute. IARC has designated RF radiation as a category 2B carcinogen. Hypotheses of reproductive or teratogenic effects have not been verified.

A283. (b). Best fit. Mobile phones operate within the microwave end of the RF spectrum. The mechanism by which RF: EMF radiation affects the male reproductive system has not yet been elucidated. Some epidemiological studies have found increased rates of both acoustic neuroma and brain cancers, but inconsistent results preclude the drawing of conclusions at this time.

A284. (b). Best fit. Non-ionising radiation incorporates radio frequency (RF) radiation (including microwaves), infrared, visible radiation and ultraviolet.

A285. (c). Best fit. Visible radiation (light) lies between the infrared and ultraviolet portion of the electromagnetic spectrum. The retina is most sensitive to blue light (400–750 nm) and damage may be structural, thermal or photochemical. Lasers can cause pressure-induced (mechanical) retinal damage as well as thermal. Individuals with aphakia (but not cataracts) are more susceptible to retinal damage and should wear spectacle filters when working in bright environments. Glare and insufficient lighting can cause eye strain, eye irritation, visual fatigue and headache which is more likely in those over 40 years of age. Symptoms are transient.

A286. (b). The typical latent period is six to eight hours but can be as little as one hour with very high exposure. It is caused UVB and UVC but not infrared or UVA. Lid chemosis is common as is punctate ulceration which may be coalescent on fluorescein staining.

A287. (e). Best fit. Lasers are classified with increasing energy from 1 to 4. The Class 4 is the most dangerous as it has most energy. Class 1 lasers are used in pointers and are relatively safe. Class 2 lasers would require prolonged exposure to do damage. Class 3R have energies of 1 mW to 4.99 mW but 3B from 5 mW to 499 mW.

A288. (a). Prolonged IR exposure can lead to lens, cornea and retina damage, including cataracts, corneal ulcers and retinal burns. To help protect against long-term IR exposure, workers can wear personal protective equipment with IR filters or reflective coatings. One of the issues is that the worker rarely complains of symptoms such as pain at the time of exposure.

A289. (c). Best fit. An electric field is produced by voltage. As the voltage increases, the electric field increases in strength. Electric fields are measured in volts per metre (V/m). A magnetic field results from the flow of current through wires or electrical devices and increases in strength as the current increases. Electric fields are produced whether or not a device is turned on but are shielded by walls, for example, whereas magnetic fields are produced only when current is flowing, which usually requires a device to be turned on.

A290. (e). EMF is a form of non-ionising radiation and should not be confused with ionising radiation, which is potentially more harmful. Many sources, such as electrical lighting and wiring to sockets, are trivial and present no risk.

Respiratory Disorders

A291. (c). Serial peak flow recording is a useful diagnostic aid when occupational asthma is suspected and should take place over a period of at least four weeks with one week away from the workplace.

A292. (b). Variation of greater than 20% on the serial peak flow record is the criterion used in the assessment of occupational asthma.

A293. (e). It is a fungus and reproduces up to 55°C and can survive up to 70°C. It can cause an aspergilloma in an immunocompetent person with a lung cavity such as from old tuberculosis. It is ubiquitous. Allergic bronchopulmonary aspergillosis can be treated with oral corticosteroids, sometimes used with anti-fungal medications such as itraconazole.

A294. (a). Silicosis: Soapstone is a natural stone (also known as steatite) that consists primarily of talc. It has become increasingly popular in the manufacture of kitchen countertops. It has a high silica content which produces large amounts of respirable silica when cut/sanded and has been associated with outbreaks of silicosis in workshops with poor ventilation/low-grade personal protective equipment.

A295. (b). COPD: This worker is a lifelong smoker with a hyperinflated chest X-ray, which would suggest air trapping and therefore an obstructive lung condition. COPD remains common (and underdiagnosed) and should be considered in anyone over 35 years of age with a significant smoking history or with evidence of other health conditions which are smoking related. Pleural plaques are a sign of asbestos exposure but in themselves, plaques do not cause significant respiratory symptoms. Asbestosis is the pulmonary fibrosis associated with significant asbestos exposure and as with other fibrotic conditions (silicosis and IPF) produce fine 'Velcro' crackles on examination. Mesothelioma typically presents with pain, breathlessness and evidence of a new pleural effusion or pleural thickening.

A296. (b). Laboratory animal allergy is common in those who carry out animal research. Respiratory Sensitisation is often seen in those working with mice, rats, guinea pigs and dogs. The allergens causing sensitisation are high molecular weight compounds commonly found in the animal's urine, which can then aerosolise when the urine dries. Handling the animals, cleaning or changing the bedding results in respiratory exposure, which can produce conjunctivitis, rhinitis and occupational asthma.

A297. (c). Peak flow monitoring: Bakers are exposed to many respiratory sensitisers in the workplace: wheat proteins, enzymes (including alpha amylase) and rye flour proteins. Many supermarkets now have bakery sections, which bake semi-manufactured bread so exposures to non–'scratch bakers' have increased significantly. Ultimately, to diagnose occupational asthma you still need to document evidence of asthma. Periods of peak flow monitoring in and away from the workplace are still required to firm up the diagnosis before any recommendations of removing workers/changing work allocations should be given.

A298. (c). Mushrooms: Mushroom workers typically will present with Hypersensitivity pneumonitis rather than asthma. Processed meats are often bulked with wheat containing rusks while coffee can produce respiratory sensitisation.

A299. (e). Bronchiolitis obliterans ('popcorn lung'): Bronchiolitis obliterans is a progressive lung condition, which produces inflammation and scarring of the smallest airways in the lungs just before the alveoli. This can occur in many conditions (most commonly as a manifestation of graft versus host disease post lung and other transplants). This bronchiolitis produces profound air flow obstruction and is progressive and irreversible often leading to lung transplantation. An outbreak in a microwave popcorn factory was found to be due to a chemical, diacetyl, found in the sweet flavouring of the popcorn. Although banned in the EU this flavouring can still be found in some of the 'sweet' flavours of vaping liquid manufactured in other countries or in unregulated vaping fluid manufacture.

A300. (a). Emphysema in cadmium workers: Cadmium is a well-recognised cause of emphysema.

A301. (b). Pneumococcal vaccine in welders: Exposure to high levels of welding fume has been shown to significantly increase the risk of pneumonia. The UK Health and Safety Executive recommends pneumococcal vaccination in workers exposed to high levels of fume despite relevant occupational hygiene mitigation measures.

A302. (d). Ammonia is an irritant, which can produce respiratory symptoms. All the others are respiratory sensitisers.

A303. (d). OASYS score = 3.5: OASYS is a statistical computer programme that plots and interprets serial peak expiratory flow (PEF) readings of patients suspected as having occupational asthma or work-related asthma. The computer-generated score has a 94% specificity for occupational asthma diagnosis and a 75% sensitivity and is seen as a standard of care in the diagnosis of occupational asthma. The scoring system runs from 1 to 4 with a score greater than 2.5 having a sensitivity of 75% of having true occupational asthma.

A304. (e). A fall in the predicted FVC below 80% should merit further investigation as per the UK Health and Safety Executive's spirometry guidance.

A305. (d). Vehicle paint technicians: According to reporting to the surveillance database SWORD, vehicle paint technicians are the most commonly seen occupation with asthma followed by bakers and flour confectioners (UK Health and Safety Executive work-related asthma statistics).

A306. (c). RADS is a form of irritant-induced airflow obstruction producing asthma-like symptoms. It is typically induced by a very significant one-off exposure to a high concentration of a respiratory irritant. It can, however, produce chronic symptoms.

A307. (e). Occupational asthma: Cockroaches are a common respiratory sensitiser producing an IgE-mediated inflammatory response (to allergens Bla g 4 and Bla g 5) which can cause occupational asthma.

A308. (e). All the others are associated with an increased risk of lung cancer except cadmium. Cadmium is a recognised cause of emphysema.

A309. (a). Hypersensitivity pneumonitis (extrinsic allergic alveolitis) is caused by a significant number of allergens. Acute hypersensitivity pneumonitis is associated with significant systemic symptoms of fever and so forth as well as respiratory symptoms. Bacterial overgrowth of metal working fluid (often with pseudomonas or mycobacterial species) is a common cause. The fluid is commonly collected in a sump and subsequently recycled throughout the work area with the result that it can often produce outbreaks leading to symptoms in multiple workers.

A310. (b). The cold environment can exacerbate underlying asthma as well as provoke 'exercise-induced bronchosconstriction'. The ice resurfacer machines which replete the ice on the rinks (are commonly fuelled by fossil fuels leading to production of carbon monoxide and nitrogen dioxide which in poorly ventilated arenas has led to symptoms of poisoning in staff and competitors.

A311. (c). Acetyl in popcorn sweeteners can cause bronchiolitis obliterans. This causes a progressive and irreversible lung disease. All the others are recognised causes of HP.

A312. (c). Bleach cleaning products produce irritant-induced asthma symptoms. All the others are respiratory sensitisers, which can produce asthma.

A313. (a). Soldering fluxes are a well-recognised cause of occupational asthma. Colophony is a biological product derived from the sap of pine trees and can act as a sensitising agent producing asthma. There are colophony-free solder fluxes, but in repair shops exposure to old colophony can still occur. Isocyanates can also be produced in the soldering process, so it is important to consider other potential causes particularly in the setting of a negative inhalation challenge. Beryllium causes a granulomatous interstitial lung disease similar to sarcoidosis. Stainless steel can produce asthma but is not associated with soldering.

A314. (c). This worker has clear occupational asthma with evidence of sensitisation, asthma and work relatedness (confirmed by peak flow monitoring). Any exposure, irrespective of the workplace exposure limits or personal protective equipment can produce/worsen symptoms leading to long-term morbidity. The only option here is redeployment.

A315. (e). This worker has significant silica exposure as well as a very significant smoking history. Long-term silica exposure and smoking have an additive effect on the risk of lung cancer development. Although significant chronic lung disease can lead to cachexia and pulmonary fibrosis can lead to clubbing, the presence of persistent haemoptysis is much more suggestive of a more sinister pathology.

A316. (e). COPD is typically caused by inhalation of dusts, gases and vapours which produces inflammation in the airways and/or structural damage to the lung. The main risk remains smoking, though smoking and working in higher risk occupations (e.g., welding) can have an additive effect. Studies which excluded smokers and those with a history of asthma have found that all of the above workers had an increased risk of developing COPD.

A317. (c). Hypersensitivity pneumonitis (hot tub lung). The clue to this is the presentation with fevers. Very few non-infective conditions will produce fevers and the symptoms described are classical for acute hypersensitivity pneumonitis. Exposure that is more prolonged can produce chronic hypersensitivity pneumonitis, which results in the development of pulmonary fibrosis. Hot tub lung develops due to a hypersensitivity reaction to a non– mycobacterium tuberculous often found in hot tubs and pools which are not adequately cleaned (or because the cleaning solutions do not eliminate the mycobacterium) with the bacteria aerosolised in the environment around the pool.

A318. (d). Asbestos exposure can produce pleural plaques, which are a painless and benign marker. Asbestosis is the pulmonary fibrosis associated with relatively high levels of asbestos exposure. Mesothelioma can develop following any (even trivial) asbestos exposure. It typically presents with pain (which can proceed any radiological evidence of pleural effusions or pleural thickening), breathlessness and weight loss. Any pleural effusion in those with evidence of pleural plaques should be considered at high risk of mesothelioma. Asbestos also increases the risk of primary lung cancer, which can present with similar symptoms.

A319. (c). Best fit. Para-phenylamine diamine-based dyes can produce contact dermatitis. Hairspray/perfumes can aggravate underlying asthma. Henna is a plant-based dye, which very rarely can cause sensitisation and asthma.

A320. (e). Coal dust is less fibrogenic than silica but can produce a nodular and fibrotic condition of coal worker's pneumoconiosis. As with any chronic exposure to dust this can increase risk of COPD, and mining can also produce respirable silica and therefore increase silicosis risk. The risk of lung cancer does not seem to be increased in coal workers, particularly those with coal worker's pneumoconiosis.

A321. (c). The most frequent acute presentation of respiratory issues in welders is metal fume fever. This produces fevers and breathlessness in response to inhalation of freshly generated zinc oxide fume. This is commonly generated from welding zinc-coated steel. Welders can get iron deposits in the lungs (welders siderosis) which gives nodular changes but not over pulmonary fibrosis.

A322. (b). Isocyanates are commonly used in the polyurethane foam in car seats as well as other vehicle parts. These low molecular weight antigens can produce sensitisation and subsequent development of occupational asthma. Immunological assays can measure the presence or concentration of these antigens.

A323. (b). Caplan syndrome, rheumatoid arthritis and coal worker's pneumoconiosis is seen in coal workers.

A324. (d). Occupational asthma remains poorly recognised by healthcare professionals.

Skin Disorders

A325. (e). Use of these creams may raise general skin hygiene awareness within a workforce. Barrier creams may in themselves be a source of contact dermatitis in some sensitive individuals. It may be true if an individual is faced with moving to a less well-paid job in order to avoid contact with an antigen. In other words, the employee is likely to remain exposed rather than accept financial loss.

A326. (e). Solvents used in this manner are a major cause of dermatitis. Treatment advised as necessary, and advice given as to how further exposure can be avoided or reduced. It is not necessary in all cases to seek alternative work if, for example, certain agents can be substituted with less irritant or non-allergenic substances. A policy should cover good personal hygiene and providing good washing facilities and appropriate protective clothing.

Non-ionic are the least likely. Excessive use of skin cleansers should be avoided as they dry the skin.

A327. (d). Rarely associated with itch. Psoriatic arthropathy is not associated with presence of rheumatoid factor in the serum. May be aggravated by physical or chemical trauma. The Koebner phenomenon is the appearance of lesions at the site of local trauma. If it involves exposed arms/forearms/scalp with shedding of scales which may be a source of staphylococcal infection.

A328. (b). Confirmation of photoallergy is by photo patch testing. The pathophysiology is similar to allergic contact dermatitis. Photoallergic skin reactions are less common than phototoxic reactions and their appearance is usually sudden. They may appear in non–sun-exposed areas.

A329. (c). Patch testing is used in the evaluation of allergic contact dermatitis and is read over the course of a week, typically on day 3 and day 5 after the patches are applied. Scarring may occur in 1 in 10,000 patch tests.

A330. (d). Best fit. The phenomenon has not been described in pityriasis rosea, a condition of unknown aetiology characterised by a 'herald patch'. Psoriasis is the most studied condition exhibiting the phenomenon in which it seems particularly prevalent in unstable psoriasis, those with young age of onset, those who have received multiple treatments for psoriasis and in winter compared with summer. It is also more prevalent in emotionally distressed individuals but is not related to the severity of the underlying skin disease. The pathogenesis remains obscure.

A331. (c). Definitive treatment of ACD is allergen avoidance. Topical corticosteroids are often used for symptom control.

A332. (c). Best fit. Transplant patients have 60 to 250 times the rate of SSC compared with general population. The high rate of SCC is felt to be related to use of immunosuppressants and sun exposure.

Institution of Occupational Safety and Health estimated the attributable fraction as 2% across males and females. Pott's famous paper was 1775 not 1875. Arsenic does cause Bowen's carcinoma *in situ* and although worldwide food and water are probably the most common exposure route, in industry inhalation and skin exposure are important. UVA does penetrate more deeply but UVB is higher energy and more likely to cause damage and carcinogenesis.

A333. (d).

A334. (c). Also known as oil acne. Can be caused by oils, pitch and tar. Greatest number due to contact with mineral oils.

A335. (e). Use of a Wood's lamp may help detect early cases.

A336. (b).

A337. (a). Chloracne is a specific form of oil acne. The causative agents are known as 'chloracnegens'. Get cystic skin lesions with comedones, principally of the face and neck.

A338. (d). Irritants may be strong (e.g., acids, alkalis, solvents) or weak (e.g., domestic detergents, oils, greases).

A339. (c). Standard batteries of antigens are used which include the suspect antigen.

A340. (e). Also known as a sensitiser. They elicit a type 4 immunological reaction.

A341. (b). An example would be coal tar pitch and sunlight.

A342. (a). Occurs rapidly on application of substances to the skin (e.g., persulphates in hairdressing). May or may not have an immunological component to its aetiology. Heat, cold, mild trauma and sunlight may be a cause in some individuals.

A343. (b). Some individuals with pre-existing non-occupational skin disease may present as part of a 'cluster' of skin problems. Occupational vitiligo may occur in clusters.

Toxicology, Metals and Solvents

A344. (a). Best fit. Evidence for adverse effects on exposed personnel is scarce and inconsistent. Further studies are needed. Halothane is scarcely used and has been largely replaced with safer alternatives (e.g., sevoflurane).

A345. (e). Best fit. In general, trivalent arsenic compounds are considered to be more toxic than pentavalent compounds. Inorganic arsenic is generally considered to be more toxic than organic form. Crustaceans and other fish are a known source of organic arsenic exposure; however, in this form, the toxicity is considered to be negligible. Estimates are that 60% to 90% of inorganic arsenic is absorbed through the gastrointestinal tract, with initial distribution predominantly going to the liver, kidney, muscle and skin. Respiratory and parenteral routes may also absorb arsenic. Dermal penetration of intact skin has not been shown to pose a risk for acute toxicity secondary to poor absorption by the integumentary system.

A346. (c). A teratogen is a chemical that causes birth defects, and a mutagen is a chemical that damages chromosomes.

A347. (d). HF exposure results in hypocalcemia, hyperkalemia, metabolic acidosis. Treatment is with calcium gluconate.

A348. (c). The LD50 is the lethal concentration of an aerosol, gas, vapour or particulate that, when administered to a group of test animals by inhalation, causes death in 50% of those animals.

A349. (d). Benzene is an aromatic organic compound.

A350. (e). Polyvinyl chloride (PVC or vinyl) is a high strength thermoplastic material widely used in applications, such as pipes, medical devices, wire and cable insulation. It is the world's third-most widely produced synthetic plastic polymer.

A351. (c). Threshold refers to the dose below which the probability of an individual responding is 0. Option 'a' is the no observable effect level, option 'b' is the latency period, option 'd' is the LD50, and option 'e' is the biologic gradient.

A352. (d). Best fit. The unique properties of NP have led to a scientific and technological explosion, albeit they have always been present in the environment. An NP has all three dimensions in the nanoscale (1 nm to 100 nm). They can be synthesised by a 'top-down' (grinding or lithography) or a 'bottom-up' (chemical synthesis) approach. Their unique characteristics influence their chemical reactivity as well as their mechanical, optical, electrical and magnetic properties. Free-engineered NP and nanomaterials are more likely to pose risk to human health and the environment than nanostructured objects (e.g., microprocessor chips).

A353. (c). Occur by the process of evaporation at a solid or liquid surface.

A354. (a). The change is often associated with a chemical change (e.g., oxidation). Fume particles may be very fine (i.e., less than 1 μm).

A355. (d). May form as the result of splashing, atomising or foaming. Examples are mists from cutting/grinding oils.

A356. (b).

A357. (d). Amino levalunic acid. Blood lead is used more frequently as a biological monitor.

A358. (c). Urinary metabolite used for biological monitoring.

A359. (a). Urinary metabolite used for biological monitoring.

A360. (e). Urinary metabolite used for biological monitoring.

A361. (b).

A362. (d). Also raised blood lead levels.

A363. (a). Erethism is a toxic organic psychosis.

A364. (e).

A365. (b).

A366. (c).

A367. (b). Green discoloration of the tongue is an indication of exposure to vanadium but not necessarily of toxicity.

A368. (e). Elemental vanadium is rare in nature. Vanadium pentoxide is considered a possible but not probable a human carcinogen but is rarely linked with hepatic or renal toxicity.

A369. (b). Best fit. Secondary aluminium smelting processes have previously been found to be important sources of polychlorinated dibenzo-p-dioxins (PCDDs) and polychlorinated dibenzofurans (PCDFs). Recycling of aluminium involves melting the scrap metal at very high temperatures and casting to form new ingots. The potential for PCDD/F exposure of employees at recycling plants is well recognised and regulations are usually in place to control exposure. The Hall–Héroult process releases carbon dioxide. Whilst bauxite can be contaminated with various trace elements, including beryllium, a significant risk of respiratory problems is not recognised. Telangiectasia is documented as being found in aluminium smelting workers whilst a direct relationship with cardiovascular disease is not.

A370. (b). Best fit. Cadmium is found in cigarettes with high levels linked to adverse health effects like chronic obstructive pulmonary disease. Smokers have higher cadmium concentrations in their blood compared with non-smokers. Smoking creates cadmium oxide, which is absorbed into the body through the lungs. Cadmium is recognised as a Group 1 carcinogen by IARC. The excretion of cadmium is slow, which is why it accumulates, and it is partly related to the fact that the metallothionein complex is almost completely resorbed in the renal tubules.

A371. (d). Elemental mercury is not an essential element. It has a high vapour pressure and is not efficiently absorbed by ingestion. It is poorly absorbed in the gastrointestinal tract.

A372. (d). Adverse health effects are usually due to the Cr VI compounds. It is a hard silver metal. Biological monitoring is usually by post-shift measurement of Cr in urine. Inhaled chromium (VI) is a human carcinogen, resulting in an increased risk of lung cancer.

A373. (d). Best fit. Hexavalent chromium salts are irritant, corrosive and carcinogenic. Nasal perforation is usually due to inhalation of chrome vapours (e.g., chrome plating tanks). Chromium compounds are sensitisers and may cause contact dermatitis and occupational asthma. Urinary chromium measurement at the end of shifts is routinely used to measure exposure in workers.

A374. (b). One methyl group added to a benzyl ring.

A375. (a). Best fit. It is an aromatic hydrocarbon with a benzyl ring.

A376. (d). Best fit. It is somewhat more irritant but otherwise relatively similar to toluene to which it is structurally related. It is well absorbed through the skin and not a confirmed carcinogen. It forms a much lower constituent of petrol as compared with toluene.

A377. (c). A stochastic event is a random event where the probability increases with increasing exposure and has no threshold. A non-stochastic event has the severity increasing with increasing exposure and may have a threshold. Many teratogens have a threshold.

Modified Essay Questions (MEQs)

A378. The possible diagnoses are:

- Anaphylaxis.
- Syncope.
- Anxiety.
- Asthma.

A379. Anaphylaxis is a systemic allergic reaction with the potential to be life threatening if not dealt with quickly and appropriately. Typical symptoms include:

- Acute onset.
- Dyspnoea, respiratory distress, wheeze.
- Cyanosis.
- Tachycardia, hypotension.
- Urticaria, angioedema, skin changes.
- Anaphylaxis typically involves more than one symptom in more than one part of the body at the same time.

A380. Check airway breathing and circulation. If unconscious place them in the recovery position before administering adrenaline and performing CPR if necessary. Ensure that they are lying down and call for assistance. Administer adrenaline into the lateral thigh as soon as possible: 500 mcg (0.5 ml of 1:1,000) IM.

A381. Administer a further dose of adrenaline into the lateral thigh as soon as possible. 500 mcg (0.5 ml of 1:1,000) IM. Consider adrenaline again after five minutes if there has been no improvement. Also consider chlorphenamine 10 mg IM or IV or hydrocortisone 200 mg IM or IV.

A382. The patient should be brought to the emergency department for assessment and observation. A biphasic allergic reaction can occur from 1 hour to 72 hours after the initial reaction, where the symptoms of anaphylaxis occur immediately and then recur up to 72 hours later. Treatment is the same emergency medical treatment. If the diagnosis is in doubt, consider taking blood samples for mast cell tryptase. The absence of an elevated level does not exclude anaphylaxis.

A383. Isocyanate exposure from two pack spray paints. Isocyanates are commonly found in automotive paints. The major route of occupational exposure to isocyanates is inhalation of the vapour or aerosol.

A384. Respiratory sensitisation and occupational asthma. Occupational asthma symptoms may include wheeze, cough, shortness of breath and chest tightness as well as upper respiratory symptoms such as rhinitis and eye itching. Isocyanates are also very irritant, and exposure can also result in hypersensitivity pneumonitis.

Symptoms typically get worse on return to work and go away during weekends and leave.

The longer the ongoing exposure to the agent the more likely there will be permanent asthma symptoms.

A385. Hierarchy of control: elimination or substitution of the isocyanate with a less harmful product technical measures such as enclosure, isolation of the spray-painting area, local exhaust ventilation, general ventilation, job rotation, personal protective equipment.

Also monitoring of the airborne concentration, provision of information and training, keeping of records and provision of health surveillance.

A386. Typical health surveillance for occupational asthma would include a pre-employment assessment with pulmonary function testing and periodic pulmonary function testing at a minimum of three months after commencing the task and then annually. This should be accompanied by the completion of a validated questionnaire to detect symptoms of asthma or respiratory sensitisation (including rhinitis and itchy eyes as well as lower respiratory symptoms).

A387. The following may be useful:

- Medical history.
- Occupational history, smoking history, family history.
- Clinical examination.
- Lung function testing.
- Serial peak flow testing.
- Skin prick testing and blood testing for allergens.
- Bronchial challenge test.

A388. The following are examples:

- Animal handlers and animal proteins.
- Bakers and grain or amylase.
- Metal workers and cobalt.

- Furniture manufacturers and wood dust or formaldehyde.
- Healthcare workers and latex.

A389. Avoiding the workplace substance that causes symptoms is essential. Once sensitised to a substance even tiny amounts may trigger asthma symptoms, even if wearing personal protective equipment. Stopping smoking is also advised if applicable.

A390. Headache and mucous membrane irritation.

A391. The physical factors are:

- Central ventilation system with significant proportion of recirculated air.
- Air-conditioning system.
- Increased room temperature.
- Perceived and actual dryness of indoor air (low relative humidity).

A392. Initial questions include:

- What type of complaints and their frequency and distribution.
- HR data: sickness absence levels, staff turnover, staff complaints, employee satisfaction surveys, industrial relations issues.
- Review of safety statement.
- Review of organisational structure.
- Work patterns (e.g., shifts) and processes (maintenance, refurbishment, cleaning).

A393. Potential chemical air contaminants include:

- Formaldehyde: may evaporate from resins in particle board and plywood.
- Volatile organic compounds (VOCs): may evaporate from carpet glues and drying paint. New computers may also emit low levels of VOCs.
- Ozone: as well as VOCs and hydrocarbons, and dust from paper and toner may be emitted by photocopiers.
- Dust: increased levels of dust in the environment have been associated with increased reporting of symptoms.

A394. Mechanical back pain.

A395. Current symptoms of interest would include:

- Night pain.
- Constitutional symptoms (fever, weight loss).
- Bladder or bowel dysfunction.

A396. Important elements of medical history would include:

- Previous cancer.
- Previous steroid therapy or previously diagnosed osteoporosis.
- Recent bacterial infection.

A397. The following yellow flags are worth discussion:

- Belief that back pain is harmful and seriously disabling.
- Fear-avoidance behaviour and reduced activity levels.
- Tendency to low mood and social withdrawal.
- Expectation that passive treatments will help rather than belief in active participation.

A398. Yes: evidence of both. Whole leg giving way is a behavioural symptom and the bracing of her loin as well as the grimacing and sighing are signs of overt pain behaviour.

A399. Yes: these include positive axial loading, non-anatomical or superficial tenderness, distracted straight leg raise discrepancy.

A400. No investigations indicated.

A401. Consider NSAIDs at lowest effective dose for shortest period (considering need for gastro-protection). If contraindicated, not tolerated or ineffective, consider weak opioid with or without paracetamol. Paracetamol alone is not appropriate in this setting (NICE 2016). Heat packs also useful. Encourage normal activity and early return to modified work.

A402. These diseases are:

- Hepatitis B.
- Hepatitis C.
- HIV.

A403. The following is the suggested management:

- Urgent first aid.
- Initial wound care.
- Decide if a significant exposure has occurred.
- Check if the recipient is immune to hepatitis B. Check if the recipient has a history of either hepatitis B or C, or HIV infection.
- Try to get the following source bloods:
  - Hepatitis B surface Antigen:HBsAg.
  - Antibody to hepatitis C: anti-HCV.
  - HIV Antigen and Antibody:HIV Ag/Ab.
- Complete a risk assessment of the exposure.
- Decide on actions to be taken.
  - Hepatitis B PEP.
  - HIV PEP.
  - Follow-up bloods at six weeks and three months.
  - Support: Psychological.

A404. The diseases and timeline are as follows:

- Hepatitis B: Hepatitis B vaccine is highly effective in preventing acute infection after exposure if given within seven days and preferably withing 48 hours. Hepatitis B immunoglobulin (HBIG) is only indicated where the source is known HBsAg Positive, or where the recipient is a known non responder to hepatitis B vaccine AND the source is known to be high risk. HBIG should ideally be given within 48 hours but not later than seven days after exposure.
- HIV: Post-exposure prophylaxis should be considered only if within 72 hours of the exposure.

A405. The differential diagnoses are active TB and latent TB.

A406. Try to rule out active TB by arranging a chest X-ray and performing a clinical examination to include a detailed history of any relevant symptoms of TB, for example:

- Night sweats.
- Unintentional weight loss.
- Haemoptysis.
- New cough longer than three weeks' duration.
- Fever.
- Fatigue.
- Chills.
- Loss of appetite.
- Chest pain.

A407. The implications are as follows:

- If the diagnosis is latent TB infection, then there is no impact on the HCW's fitness for duty as the condition is not infectious to others.
- The HCW should be offered treatment for the latent TB infection. The HCW is not compelled to take the treatment offered. If treatment is declined, follow-up surveillance should be arranged as per national guidelines.
- If the diagnosis is active TB, then the HCW is unfit for duty as the condition is infectious to others. The HCW should be referred to a respiratory specialist and deemed unfit for duty until such time as the condition is treated and deemed no longer infectious by the respiratory specialist.

A408. The following outlines the initial management:

- Medical history, concentrating on history of illness that may impact hearing.
- Occupational history for noise exposure and head trauma or ototoxic agent exposure, including medication use.
- Relevant family history.
- Social history of recreational exposure to noise.
- Functional assessment of hearing during the consultation.
- Assessment of impact of tinnitus.

A409. The following investigations/assessments will be useful:

- Examination of the external and internal structure of the ears.
- Hearing test carried out in soundproof booth.
- Referral for formal specialist audiology opinion.

A410. The following should be considered:

- Noise-induced occupational hearing loss.
- Noise-induced non-occupational hearing loss.
- Age-related hearing loss alone or in combination with the above.
- Any or all of the above combined with tinnitus.

A411. The hierarchy of control is applicable:

- Elimination or substitution of the noise hazard.
- Control of the noise at source by technical measures such as enclosure, isolation of the source, maintenance procedures.
- Control of transmission by acoustic barriers and tiles, distancing, rotation of staff to decrease overall exposure duration.
- Protection of operators by use of appropriate personal protective equipment, isolation behind enclosures.

A412. The following measures are important:

- Monitoring of noise levels.
- Information and training of staff on risk from noise and on appropriate control measures.
- Consultation with staff.
- Evidence of record-keeping and reporting.
- Health surveillance to include the use of an appropriate noise questionnaire and periodic audiometry.

A413. Advice would include education about hearing, reducing exposure to loud noise, use of hearing protection, use of hearing amplification and making sure that follow-up, including hearing tests, is arranged. The importance of avoiding further excessive noise exposure from all sources, at home and at work. The importance of adhering to the protective measures provided by the employer, including personal protective measures. An explanation of the exponential mechanism of harm resulting from noise and the ability to accumulate a dose in short periods of time when the noise level is loud. Arrangements for health surveillance.

A414. The most likely diagnosis is contact irritant dermatitis (as the web spaces are preferentially affected). Other diagnoses include contact allergic dermatitis (less likely); worsening of pre-existing eczema, depending on past medical history; dyshidrotic eczema—check between the toes for tinea pedis and possible id reaction; psoriasis—less likely but possibly a Koebner-type reaction.

A415. The most likely diagnosis is contact irritant dermatitis. In nurses this is typically due to repeated hand washing, contact with soaps and alcohol, maceration from glove use, irritation from contact with bedsheets. A work-related cause is suggested if the hands and exposed skin are affected if the condition improves away from work and relapses on return and if more than one person is affected in the work area. The effect of an irritant depends on several factors, including how irritant the substance is, the concentration and duration of exposure.

Certain people seem to be more sensitive to irritants, including those with childhood eczema, atopy, very dry skin and those with very fair complexions. There may be a contact allergy component, and this may typically be due to latex which can cause a type 1 or a type 4 allergy, and chlorhexidine which can result in a type 4 allergy. Glove allergy to chemical constituents of gloves is also a possibility-due to accelerators., antioxidants, (thiurams, carbamates). Possible combined irritant and allergic contact dermatitis. An irritant contact dermatitis may develop first, and this may make the skin more susceptible to sensitisation and an allergic contact dermatitis might be later maintained by exposure to an irritant.

A416. The following are applicable:

- First, take a detailed history and perform a skin examination.
- Medical history, concentrating on history of skin problems, sensitivity, allergy and atopy, hay fever, eczema and asthma.
- History of anaphylaxis to other latex-containing products.
- Occupational history for chemical and glove exposure and including medication use family history of skin problems and allergies.
- Social history for exposure to irritants and allergens.
- Full skin examination to look for psoriasis, tinea pedis, line of demarcation suggesting a glove reaction.

A417. The following are applicable:

- Review the risk assessment.
- Implement a hierarchy of control approach to the risk and review control measures to determine their effectiveness.
- Elimination or substitution of the offending irritants.
- Technical measures such as enclosure, isolation, job rotation, personal protective equipment.
- Provision of information and training, keeping of records and provision of health surveillance.

A418. The lack of improvement suggests that other factors such as an allergic component need to be considered. In addition, a more potent steroid may be required with intensifications of the skin care regime. If type 1 allergy is suspected, consider blood testing for allergens. If type 4 contact allergy is suspected, then consider referral for patch testing. A period of time away from the workplace and avoiding all contact with suspect agents may need to be considered. The skin is a slow-growing organ, and a process of relapse remission is not uncommon if protective measures are not adhered to completely or for long enough. Also, it is important to review any non-work-related exposures as these often contribute to the maintenance of the skin problem.

A419. The most common cause of occupational dermatitis is contact irritant dermatitis, and this usually resolves with a combination of removing exposure from the offending agents as well as an appropriate skin care regime aimed at improving the skin integrity and the waxy outer layer of the stratum corneum. Avoiding the workplace substance that causes symptoms is essential. Often a number of agents may be at fault, and it may be that removal from the workplace is required for a period of time. It is also necessary to consider whether a combination of irritation and allergy is causing the problem in which case referral to a contact dermatitis clinic should be considered.

General advice on skin care will always include appropriate use of emollients. If there is an inflammatory element, then a short-term course of moderate to potent steroids may be helpful. It is essential to review the protective equipment used and to ensure that the appropriate gloves are used for the appropriate exposure while acknowledging that in certain cases the gloves themselves maybe contributing to the problem either by causing maceration of the skin with prolonged glove use or allergy to a component of the glove. Appropriate use of protective equipment at work and at home is essential as it is not uncommon for non-work-related exposure to agents such as shampoos, conditioners, and polishes can cause or exacerbate the situation. Once sensitised to a substance even tiny amounts may trigger symptoms, even if wearing protective equipment.

A420. The three categories are as follows:

- Simple mechanical back pain.
- Disc-related or radicular pain.
- Serious underlying pathology (e.g., cancer, infection, trauma or inflammatory disease such as spondyloarthritis).

A421. Simple mechanical back pain.

A422. The following is applicable:

- Provide advice and information, tailored to his needs and capabilities, to help him self-manage his low back pain.
- An anti-inflammatory medication at the lowest effective dose.
- Consider weak opioids (with or without paracetamol) for managing acute low back pain only if an NSAID is contraindicated, not tolerated or has been ineffective.
- Gentle mobilisation and exercises.

A423. The following is applicable:

- Promote and facilitate return to work or normal activities of daily living for people with low back pain with or without sciatica.
- Unfit for duty that involves tasks that aggravate the reported pain.
- Suggest modified duty as a reasonable accommodation.
- Avoid high-risk manual handling as may be identified by a manual handling risk assessment.
- Avoid static postures (i.e., prolonged sitting or standing).
- Avoid tasks that aggravate the reported symptoms such as repetitive bending and stooping.

A424. Suggest a manual handling risk assessment of the role.

A425. Work-related stress is the adverse reaction to perceived excessive pressures or other types of demands placed on an individual at work. Stress is not an illness—it is a state. However, if stress becomes too excessive and prolonged, then mental, and physical, illness may develop.

A426. The management standards cover six key areas of work design that, if not properly managed, are associated with poor health, lower productivity and increased accident and sickness absence rates. They are:

- Demands: this includes issues such as workload, work patterns and the work environment.
- Control: how much say the person has in the way they do their work.
- Support: this includes the encouragement, sponsorship and resources provided by the organisation, line management and colleagues.
- Relationships: this includes promoting positive working to avoid conflict and dealing with unacceptable behaviour.
- Role: whether people understand their role within the organisation and whether the organisation ensures that they do not have conflicting roles.
- Change: how organisational change (large or small) is managed and communicated in the organisation.

A427. The following are applicable:

- Employee Assistance Program.
- Refer to her general practitioner if clinically appropriate.
- Lifestyle advice on the following: hydration, healthy diet, good sleep, hygiene, exercise, alcohol consumption and smoking.

A428. Unfit for duty and unfit to meet with management to address perceived workplace stressors. Unfit for duty but fit to meet with management to address perceived workplace stressors.

A429. Dry eye is a condition where the surface of the eye becomes inflamed and sore due to a poor relationship between the tear film and the eyelids. This might be because the eyes are not producing enough tears or that the chemistry of the tear film is out of balance.

A430. The following are applicable:

- Eye drops/eye lubricants/eyelid wipes.
- Heat pads.
- Eye nutrition/general hydration.
- Adjust spectacles.
- Computer monitor adjustments/settings to reduce glare.
- Task lighting assessment.
- Eye exercises.
- Adjust air quality if necessary.
- Assess breaks from work.
- Consult optometry.

A431. The following are applicable:

- How does she clean the trays?
- What does she clean the trays with?
- What protection does she have?
- Does the rash improve when she is not at work?
- Has she seen her general practitioner about the rash?

A432. The following are applicable:

- Allergic contact eczema.
- Irritant contact eczema.
- Eczema due to wet work.
- New endogenous eczema.

A433. The following are applicable:

- Is the stainless steel hypoallergenic?
- Has the stainless steel been tested for nickel as not all stainless steel has nickel?
- Is the equipment very old before EU limitations on stainless steel nickel emission?
- How long is her arm in contact, and is it skin to metal?
- What is the surface cleaned with and how often?
- Does she react to other nickel sources like jewellery and coins?

A434. The following are applicable:

- General health, are they infected with any other blood-borne viruses?
- What treatment are they taking for HIV and what is their history of infection, blood results?
- What specialty do they work in or want to work in?
- Will they be performing EPPs or work in an EPP environment?
- Are they registered with UKAP-OHR, and if so, what is their registration number?
- Who is their GUM consultant, and do they have regular review?

A435. The following are applicable:

- Advise they will not be cleared for EPPs now as they have missed the window for monitoring blood tests.
- Determine why they missed their blood tests.
- Consent for HIV viral load blood tests and advised they will need repeated in 12 weeks.
- Consent to write to their previous occupational health consultant.
- Agree if you will register as the supervising occupational health consultant should they take the job.

A436. The following are applicable:

- Clarify history and medication.
- Repeat their viral load test 10 days after the original.
- If the test is less than 200 cp/m, they can continue to perform EPPs.
- If the test if still 200 cp/m or greater, then they must stop EPPs until they have two consecutive tests less than 200 cp/m no less than 12 weeks apart.
- Clarify they can continue to perform non-EPP work.

A437. The following are applicable:

- Unable to drive on ordinary driving licence for six months after single episode and unable to drive on GP2 licence for 12 months after a single episode of cough syncope.
- Needs to inform the licensing authority.

A438. The fact that her reflux has resolved does not change the period off driving. Having cough syncope indicates a predisposition to syncope with coughing from any cause.

A439. The following are applicable:

- Needs to continue the required regular monitoring of glucose.
- She cannot rely on the flash monitoring of glucose.
- For a Group 2 HGV licence, she must have full awareness of hypoglycaemia.

A440. The following are applicable:

- Unimmunised infants (born after 32 weeks) less than two months of age whose mothers did not receive pertussis vaccine after 16 weeks of pregnancy and at least two weeks prior to delivery.
- Unimmunised infants (born less than 32 weeks) less than two months of age regardless of maternal vaccine status.
- Unimmunised and partially immunised infants (fewer than three doses of vaccine) age two months and older regardless of maternal vaccine status.

A441. HCWs dealing with infants and pregnant women.

A442. HCW contacts who have not received a booster dose of pertussis vaccine more than one week and less than five years ago.

A443. Pertussis should be considered for all those offered chemoprophylaxis. HCWs who have not had vaccination in the last five years and no Td/IPV in the preceding month.

Observed Structured Practical Examination Questions (OSPEs)

A444. She has evidence of chronic hepatitis B virus (HBV) infection with the 'surface' antigen confirming natural infection. Her negative IgM core antibody suggests this is not a recent infection (albeit IgM core antibody may be present in some patients with severe exacerbation of chronic HBV infection). The fact that she is 'e' antigen negative and 'e' antibody positive suggests but does not prove that she is not highly infectious to others. These markers were previously used to show viral replication and infectivity but their use has been largely superseded by DNA. She is not co-infected with hepatitis D virus.

A445. Liver funtion tests would clarify whether she has biochemical hepatitis even if she is well. A measure of HBV DNA is a direct measure of viral load. This would determine the level of activitity of her infection and whether she might benefit from anti-viral treatment.

A446. Yes—she is fit for work.

A447. This doctor would be considered unfit to work as a general surgeon due to the potential risk posed to patients during exposure prone procedures (EPPs).

A448. The viral load is quite high and exceeds the usual threshold above which the risk of transmission of the virus to a patient, per-operatively, may occur, through inadvertent self-injury with a needle or sharp instrument.

A449. All international guidelines agree that treatment should be begun in those with HBV DNA viral load greater than 2×10^4 IU/ml.

A450. The following are applicable:

- COVID-19 re-infection.
- False Positive COVID-19 PCR result with an adverse reaction to the COVID-19 vaccine.
- False Positive COVID-19 PCR result with some other infection giving rise to the temperature and fatigue.

A451. The following are applicable:

- You would ask for a Ct value on the PCR swab result. Ct (cycle threshold) values represent the number of cycles of amplification elapsed before the test system signals detection of the target. In general terms, the higher

the Ct value the lower the quantity of virus target present in the sample. Precise definition of what constitutes a high or very high Ct value is difficult because a Ct value is not comparable to the quantitative output from a calibrated assay. The Ct value for a given sample will be different in different laboratories depending on the test platform. In general terms a Ct value of 30 or greater is considered a high Ct value and a value of 35 or greater is considered a very high Ct value.
- If the Ct value is low, it will be consistent with a new infection.
- If the Ct value is high, it may be early in a re-infection or it may be residual non-viable RNA from the previous infection.
- You would suggest a repeat PCR swab 24 hours later if the Ct value is high. If the Ct value remains high, or is higher, it is likely to be residual non-viable RNA from the previous infection. If the Ct value is lower, it is likely to be re-infection.
- Liaise with the local consultant microbiologist for such case for a definitive diagnosis.
- Depending on the diagnosis, the HCW should follow the Public Health Guidance and Occupational Health Guidance on self-isolation requirements, fitness for duty and contact tracing requirements.

A452. The following are applicable:

- Vascular: such as skin blanching of the fingers, anaesthesia associated with blanching, a sequence of colour changing in which blanching is followed by cyanosis and redness, sometimes accompanied by pain.
- Neurological: such as numbness, tingling, elevated sensory thresholds for touch, vibration, temperature, pain.
- Musculoskeletal: such as difficulty with his grip strength, reduced dexterity, locked grip and pain.

A453. The following are applicable:

- The results of any occupational hygiene measurements in regard to the magnitude of vibration that employees are exposed to for particular tasks.
- Check if colleagues have reported similar issues.

A454. The following are applicable:

- Participation in sports, a second job, hobbies that require use of the affected upper limb.
- A previous history of the reported symptoms.
- Age, smoking status, previous traumatic injury affecting the wrist.
- Consider systemic rheumatological disorders.

A455. Restrict duty: the employee should be taken off the task until symptoms resolve. Consider reasonable accommodations—alternative tasks that do not involve manual work with the affected upper limb should be sought.

A456. Initial treatment: suggest a prescription for an over-the-counter anti-inflammatory medication such as ibuprofen.

A457. Occupational hygiene input would be useful: suggest that occupational hygiene measurements are taken to measure the magnitude of exposure to hand–arm vibration.

If the occupational hygiene measurements demonstrate a level greater than 2.5 m/s^2, then a health surveillance programme should be put in place. If the occupational hygiene measurements demonstrate a level greater than 5 m/s^2, then the employees should limit their duration on this task to ensure that the hand–arm vibration exposure is not greater than 5 m/s^2. Health and safety input would also be a consideration—suggest that the employees' technique of performing the task is assessed to ensure that he is completing the task correctly. This may involve an assessment of his hand grip.

A458. Maintain follow-up—suggest review of the employee after one week. If the employee continues to have symptoms, referral to a physiotherapist may be beneficial. If the employee continues to have symptoms after approximately four sessions of physiotherapy, an MRI of the right wrist and hand may be required.

A459. Rehabilitation back to the original task: if the symptoms settle with the treatment set out above, the employee may return to the same task in a phased manner with the direction that he should report any recurrence of symptoms in a timely manner. The return to work the same task is dependent on satisfactory occupational hygiene measurements.

A460. The following are applicable:

- Contact irritant dermatitis.
- Contact allergic dermatitis.
- Non-work-related hand dermatitis.

A461. The following are applicable:

- The site of the rash: Does the rash extend beyond exposed areas of skin?
- The time of onset: Did the rash occur prior to commencing on the ward?
- History of atopy?
- A personal history of skin rashes?
- A personal family history of skin rashes?
- Any known allergies?
- Usage of gloves, duration of glove usage per shift, any hand sweating while wearing gloves, the types of gloves used, any issue in the past with latex or rubber products or nitrile gloves?
- Hand-washing frequency during a shift, soap, moisturiser and alcohol gel hand sanitiser usage?
- Any eyelid swelling and itching?

A462. Type 4: cell-mediated immunological reaction.

A463. Type 1: immunoglobulin E (IgE)-mediated.

A464. Contact irritant dermatitis: approximately 80% of cases are contact irritant.

A465. Frequent washing and scrubbing of the skin of her hands, causing an irritant and dehydrating effect.

A466. Suggest restricting the employee from the causative factor (i.e., hand washing) until the rash resolves. Provide appropriate treatment (i.e., a moisturiser and topical steroid if necessary).

Once her skin has recovered and the rash has resolved, she may return to work with instruction and training on safe hand care (i.e., the use of alcohol gel sanitiser, designed for certain uses which would reduce the requirement for hand washing, and the use of moisturisers after hand washing to help maintain her skin health).

A467. The student nurse should be restricted from clinical duty if she has broken skin on her hands and/or forearms (e.g., fissures). This would be an infection prevention and control risk (e.g., becoming colonised or infected with MRSA and spreading it to patients).

A468. Patch testing.

A469. Shoulder complaints are reasonably common presentations to OH clinics, general practice, orthopaedic clinics and EDs. Common acute problems include fractures, dislocation of the shoulder joint and rotator cuff injuries. Common chronic problems include frozen shoulder and arthritis. The following outlines the assessment of a shoulder joint at an OSPE station.

- STEP 1: Wash your hands and introduce yourself to the patient. Clarify the patient's identity. Explain that you would like to examine the patient and obtain their consent to proceed. Expose the shoulder joint which should be from the waist up and a chaperone should be offered.
- STEP 2: INSPECTION. With the patient standing, perform a general inspection of the shoulder joint from the front, side and back. Look for symmetry, wasting, scars or obvious bony deformity.
- STEP 3: FEEL. Feel over the joint and its surrounding areas to assess the temperature. Raised temperature may indicate joint infection or inflammation.
- STEP 4: PALPATE. Systematically feel along both sides of the bony shoulder girdle. Start at the sternoclavicular joint, go along the clavicle to the acromioclavicular joint, feel the acromion, and then around the spine of the scapula. Feel the anterior and posterior joint lines of the glenohumeral joint and finally the muscles around the joint for any tenderness.
- STEP 5: ACTIVE MOVEMENT. The movements of the joint should begin by being performed actively. Ask the patient to bring their arm forward (flexion), bend their arm at the elbow and push backwards (extension). Bring their arm out to the side and up above their head (abduction). Flex the elbow and tuck it into the side and move the hand outwards (external rotation). And finally see how far they can place their hand up their back (internal rotation).

- STEP 6: PASSIVE MOVEMENT. Perform all of the above movements again passively, carefully watching the patient for any pain or discomfort. Feel for any joint crepitus on movement.
- STEP 7: SPECIAL TESTS. There are many special tests for the shoulder that are commonly carried out.
  - *The impingement test:* performed by placing the shoulder out at 90 degrees with the arm hanging down, press back on the arm and check for any pain. Assesses for impingement of supraspinatus.
  - *The apprehension test:* is similar but the arm is facing upwards and push back on the arm; the patient may be apprehensive about the movement as the joint feels unstable. Assesses the integrity of the glenohumeral joint capsule.
  - *The scarf test:* performed with the elbow flexed to 90 degrees, placing the patient's hand on their opposite shoulder, and pushing back. Again, look for any discomfort. Assesses the function of the acromioclavicular joint.
- STEP 8: FUNCTIONAL TESTS. There are two quick functional tests of the shoulder that can be carried out. These involve the patient placing their hands behind their head and behind their back. This checks that they can perform everyday tasks.
- STEP 9: Thank the patient, tell them they can dress, wash your hands and summarise your findings.

NOTE: Always compare both shoulders when carrying out an assessment.

A470. There may be no clinical findings or there may be shortness of breath, decreased air entry, cyanosis, clubbing. Generally, there will be no wheeze.

A471. This picture is that of a restrictive lung disease. Full clinical and occupational history looking for a history of exposure to agents that may cause a restrictive deficit. Consider radiology and full pulmonary work-up.

A472. Restrictive deficit associated with asbestosis, interstitial fibrosis and siderosis. In this case, the heating engineer was exposed to asbestos pipe lagging in the early years of his apprenticeship.

A473. Pleural plaques on the chest X-ray.

A474. Occupational history to establish any relevant exposures, bronchoscopy and pulmonary function testing to identify asbestosis and mesothelioma or lung carcinoma.

A475. These are benign but are a sign of asbestos exposure and there may be an increased risk of other asbestos effects. Avoid further asbestos exposure, do not smoke, get routine vaccines.

Consider periodic low-dose CT screening. In some countries pleural plaques are compensable with the relevant occupation and exposure.

A476. Noise meter.

A477. Measurement of environmental noise level. It allows quick sound-level checks of machinery noise, office noise and other issues around the workplace to be carried out. It measures the instantaneous sound level with either A- or C-weighting. Most noise regulations require A-weighting. It also has both fast and slow time response. The device needs regular calibration, and depending on the device will have a range of 30 dB (A) to 130 dB (A) or 40 dB (C) to 130 dB (C). The unit of acoustic measurement for sound is usually the decibel (dB); however, some sound-level meter devices also determine the equivalent continuous sound level (Leq) and other acoustic parameters.

A478. To protect from the effect of wind on the measurement.

A479. Performance of an audiogram (hearing test) being carried out using a soundproof booth and an operator using a manual audiometer.

A480. At pre-employment, periodically as part of a health surveillance program, post injury, at exit from jobs where excess noise exposure is a risk.

A481. Breath alcohol analyser.

A482. Measurement of breath alcohol as an estimate of blood alcohol concentration (BAC). Readings are usually in micrograms of alcohol in 100 ml of air. Reference limits are available.

A483. In line with an alcohol and substance abuse policy this may be used at pre-employment, random testing and for cause testing where alcohol use is suspected.

A484. Hand grip dynamometer or grip meter.

A485. The purpose of using a hand dynamometer is to measure the maximum isometric strength of the hand and forearm muscles. It can be adjusted for hand size and must be calibrated regularly for consistent results. Hand grip strength can be quantified by measuring the amount of static force that the hand can squeeze around a dynamometer. The force is commonly measured in kilograms and pounds, but also in millilitres of mercury and in Newtons.

A486. The subject holds the dynamometer in the hand to be tested, with the arm at right angles and the elbow by the side of the body. The handle of the dynamometer is adjusted. The subject squeezes the dynamometer with maximum isometric effort and the best result from several trials for each hand is recorded.

A487. Can be used for testing hand grip strength of athletes and others involved in strength training or participants in sports in which the hands are used for catching, throwing or lifting such as gymnasts and tennis players. In occupational settings, grip strength testing can form a part of clinical examination in the assessment of upper limb conditions. It provides a means to quantitatively assess progress through rehabilitation. Grip strength has been shown to be a predictor of future disability, morbidity and mortality in a non-clinical population. There are reference standards available.

A488.

Common presenting complaints are pain in the knee, the knee locking or the knee giving way. Common causative conditions include arthritis, ligament and/or cartilage damage or injury. The following outlines the assessment of a knee joint at an OSPE station.

- STEP 1: Wash your hands and introduce yourself to the patient. Clarify the patient's identity. Explain that you would like to examine the patient and obtain their consent to proceed. Expose both knee joints which should be from the hips down and a chaperone should be offered.
- STEP 2: INSPECTION. Ask the patient to walk and check for any sign of limping or abnormal gait or varus or valgus deformity. With the patient lying down on their back, perform a general inspection of the knee joints from the front, side and back. Look for symmetry, wasting, scars or obvious bony deformity or fixed flexion deformity. Check for any obvious popliteal swelling (e.g., a baker's cyst). Compare both sides for symmetry.
- STEP 3: FEEL. Feel over the joint and its surrounding areas to assess the temperature. Raised temperature may indicate joint infection or inflammation.
- STEP 4: PALPATE. Palpate the border of the patella for any tenderness, behind the knee for any swellings, along all the joint lines for tenderness and at the point of insertion of the patellar tendon. Tap the patella to see if there is any effusion deep to the patella.
- STEP 5: ACTIVE MOVEMENT. The movements of the joint should begin by being performed actively. Flexion—ask them to bend their knee as far as they can. Ask about pain. Extension—ask them to straighten their knee as far as they can. Ask about pain.
- STEP 6: PASSIVE MOVEMENT. Perform all of the above movements again passively, carefully watching the patient for any pain or discomfort. Feel for any knee joint crepitus on movement.
- STEP 7: SPECIAL TESTS. For cruciate ligament instability or damage. *Anterior drawer test*: Flex the knee to 90 degrees and sit on the patient's foot. Pull forward on the tibia just distal to the knee. There should be no movement. If there is movement, it suggests anterior cruciate ligament (ACL) damage. Another test for ACL damage is the *Lachman test*. *Posterior drawer test:* With the knee in the same position, observe from the side for any posterior lag of the joint, this suggests posterior cruciate ligament damage. *Collateral ligament test*: Hold the leg with the knee flexed to 15 degrees and place lateral and medial stress on the knee. Any excessive movement suggests collateral ligament damage.

- STEP 8: FUNCTIONAL TESTS. There is one quick functional test of the knees that can be carried out. This involves the patient standing and getting them to squat down as far as they can and then up again—check for pain and stiffness. This checks that they can perform everyday tasks involving the use of the knees.
- STEP 9: Thank the patient, tell them they can dress, wash your hands and summarise your findings.

NOTE: Always compare both knees when carrying out an assessment.
The *McMurray test* for meniscal damage is no longer recommended due to concerns that it may exacerbate the injury and its low diagnostic accuracy.

A489. Nail pits: defined depressions in the plate caused by shedding of nail plate cells.

A490. Psoriasis. Nail lesions occur in 90% of patients with psoriatic arthritis. The severity of psoriatic nail involvement may correlate with the extent and severity of both skin and joint disease.

A491. The following are appropriate and found in patients with psoriasis:

- Onycholysis: separation of the nail from its bed.
- Distal nail bed hyperkeratosis: Subungual hyperkeratosis is a disorder characterised by an excessive reproduction of skin cells that accumulate between the nail and the nail bed. Also involves thickening and lifting of the nail.
- Splinter haemorrhages: A splinter haemorrhage is a longitudinal, red-brown haemorrhage under a nail and looks like a wood splinter.
- Oil-drop or salmon-patch is a translucent yellow-red discolouration in the nail bed proximal to onycholysis. It reflects inflammation and can be tender.

A492. It is a lateral or transverse view of the cervico-thoracic spine.

A493. This image shows a large thoracic disc prolapse. The transverse views showed it was a large central prolapse. The man had no trauma and no history of an acute episode but had symptoms for at least six months before presenting to occupational health. Once the image was taken, he was advised to stay in hospital until he had surgical removal of the prolapsed disc a couple of days later. He made an excellent recovery.

A494. Back pain is a very common presentation at OH clinics. Common causes of back pain include arthritis, prolapsed disc and muscular injuries. Occasionally it can be the underlying cause of other conditions such as sciatica or more rarely cancer either primary or secondary. The following outlines the assessment of a back at an OSPE station.

- STEP 1: Wash your hands and introduce yourself to the patient. Clarify the patient's identity. Explain that you would like to examine the patient and obtain their consent to proceed. Expose the entire spine and the patient should undress from the waist up. A chaperone should be offered.
- STEP 2: INSPECTION. Ask the patient to stand and walk and check for any sign of limping or abnormal gait. With the patient still standing look from behind for any obvious abnormalities such as scars. Check the muscle bulk and any wasting. Note the symmetry of each side and look for any spinal deviation such as scoliosis. Assess from the side to check for the normal curvatures of the spine in particular: cervical lordosis, thoracic kyphosis, lumbar lordosis.
- STEP 3: FEEL. Feel along the entire length of the spine column.
- STEP 4: PALPATE. Palpate each spinous process checking for tenderness. Palpate the sacroiliac joints and the paraspinal muscles. Regularly ensure there is no discomfort.
- STEP 5: ACTIVE MOVEMENT. The lumbar spine flexion and extension are checked by asking the patient to try and touch their toes (flexion) and then lean backwards (extension). Lateral flexion is examined by asking the patient to run their hand down the outside of their leg. Ask about pain.
- STEP 6: SPECIAL TESTS. With the patient lying flat on the couch, perform a *Straight Leg Raise* which assesses for nerve entrapment such as sciatica. *FABER test*: screens for sacroiliac joint and hip as cause for back pain by doing FABER test or any sacroiliac tests. *Sciatic stretch test* and *femoral stretch test* may be carried out to assess sciatic and femoral nerves respectively. Measure leg length. Tests knee (L3,4), ankle (L5, S1) and plantar reflexes *(Babinski test)*. Test lower limb sensation (L4 medial foot, L5 mid dorsum of foot, S1 lateral border of foot).
- STEP 7: Thank the patient, tell them they can dress, wash your hands and summarise your findings.

A495.

This is for measuring the bideltoid distance for offshore workers that may travel in a helicopter. Shoulder breadth (bideltoid) definition is the maximum horizontal breadth across the shoulders, measured to the protrusions of the deltoid muscles. The bideltoid distance determines where the person sits in a helicopter; for example, if they are extra-broad, they will need to be placed near a Type IV exit.

A496.

All passengers travelling to offshore work locations by helicopter are required to sit in a seat where the nearest emergency exit is compatible with their body size. These helicopter passengers are measured by the width of their shoulders and those whose shoulder width is 55.9 cm or greater are classified as extra-broad (XBR). Those below 55.9 cm will be classified as 'regular'. The Civil Aviation Authority will prohibit a passenger whose body size is not compatible with the emergency exit size (not always a push-out window). A bideltoid measurement certificate can be issued.

A497. Asbestos fibres.

A498. Lung cancer, pleural plaques, mesothelioma, asbestosis, diffuse pleural thickening.

A499. Avoid further asbestos exposure, do not smoke, get routine vaccines. Adhere to regular medical follow-up.

A500. The examination should assess any respiratory (breathing) pathology that may be the cause of a patient's symptoms: shortness of breath, coughing and wheeze. Common conditions include chest infections, asthma, and chronic obstructive pulmonary disease (COPD). In this case with a history of laboratory work with animals, occupational asthma may be a consideration. The following outlines the assessment of the respiratory system at an OSPE station.

- STEP 1: Wash your hands and introduce yourself to the patient. Clarify the patient's identity. Explain that you would like to examine the patient and obtain their consent to proceed. Expose the entire chest and the patient should undress from the waist up. A chaperone should be offered.
- STEP 2: INSPECTION. The patient should be sitting up on the couch. Check if they are distressed with rapid breathing (tachypnoea), cyanosed, chest deformities. Look at the hands for any signs of clubbing or nicotine staining. Get the patient to extend their arms and cock their wrists to 90 degrees and observe the hands in this position for 30 seconds; a coarse flap may also be a sign of carbon dioxide retention. Take the pulse at the wrist—a bounding pulse may indicate carbon dioxide retention. Count the patient's respiration rate. Ask the patient to stick out their tongue (check underneath also) and note its colour, checking for anaemia or central cyanosis. Look for any use of accessory muscles such as the sternocleidomastoid muscle. Observe the chest for any deformities or scars. Include the axillae and the back.
- STEP 3: FEEL and PALPATE. Palpate for the left supraclavicular node (Virchow's node). This drains the thoracic duct so an enlarged node (Troisier sign) may suggest metastatic cancer (e.g., lung or abdominal). Now palpate the chest. First, feel between the heads of the two clavicles for the trachea. Any deviation may suggest a tumour or pneumothorax. Feel for chest expansion. Place your hands firmly on the chest wall with your thumbs meeting in the midline. Ask the patient to take a deep breath in and note the distance your thumbs move apart. Normally this should be at least 5 cm. You should measure this at the top and bottom of the lungs as well as on the back.
  - Perform percussion on both sides, comparing similar areas on both sides. You should start by tapping on the clavicle which gives an indication of the resonance in the apex. Then percuss normally for the entire lung fields. Hyperresonance may suggest a collapsed lung, whereas hyporesonance or dullness suggests consolidation such as in infection, effusion or a tumour.

  - Check for tactile vocal fremitus. Place the medial edge of your hand on the chest and ask the patient to say '99' or 'blue balloon'. Do this with your hand in the upper, middle and lower areas of both lungs. This again gives a suggestion of the constitution of the tissue deep to your hand.
- STEP 4: AUSCULTATE. For both lungs—front and back, comparing the sides to each other. Listen for any reduced breath sounds, or added sounds such as crackles, wheeze, pleural rub or rhonchi. Test vocal fremitus again.
- STEP 5: FINISH. Examine the lymph nodes in the head and neck. Start under the chin with the submental nodes, move along to the submandibular then to the back of the head at the occipital nodes. Next palpate the pre- and post-auricular nodes. Move down the cervical chain and onto the supraclavicular nodes.
- STEP 6: Thank the patient, tell them they can dress, wash your hands and summarise your findings.

A501. Briefly explain what you are going to do and get consent. Adequately expose the upper body and ensure the patient is comfortable. Position the patient standing for initial inspection of the shoulders. Ask if they have any pain before proceeding with the clinical examination. Then follow the regular protocol: inspection, feel/palpate, move: active and passive. Thank the patient and formulate your findings and summarise for the examiner or on paper if applicable.

A502. Delayed large local reaction to vaccine. A variety of such reactions has been reported with this vaccine and others. The condition may range from mild to moderate, mimicking cellulitis, and should be distinguished from the latter, obviating the need for antibiotics.

A503. Ice and/or oral antihistamine and/or topical corticosteroids are helpful as may paracetamol for any pain or fever.

A504. No. This condition is not a contraindication to further doses of vaccine. It does not necessarily recur with a second dose and is self-limiting, usually settling in three to four days. The median time from second dose of vaccine to cutaneous symptom onset tends to be shorter. The aetiology of this delayed reaction remains unclear bit is likely to be T-cell mediated.

INDEX

I

J

K

L

N

O